IMPAIRED CONSCIOUSNESS IN
TEXTS

CW01507994

Impaired consciousness is a topic lying at the intersection of science and philosophy. It encourages reflection on questions concerning human nature, the body, the soul, the mind and their relation, as well as the blurry limits between health, disease, life and death. This is the first study of impaired consciousness in the works of some highly influential Greek and Roman medical writers who lived in periods ranging from classical Greece to the Roman Empire in the second century CE. Andrés Pelavski explores the notion and contrasts ancient and contemporary theoretical frameworks in order to challenge some established ideas about mental illness in antiquity. All the ancient texts are translated and the theoretical concepts clearly explained.

ANDRÉS D. PELAVSKI holds a postdoctoral position at the Hebrew University of Jerusalem. He is a consultant anaesthetist as well as a classicist and the book originated in his doctoral thesis at the University of Cambridge, which was awarded the Hare Prize in 2022.

CAMBRIDGE CLASSICAL STUDIES

General editors

J. P. T. CLACKSON, G. BETEGH, S. CUOMO, S. P. OAKLEY,
J. C. QUINN, M. J. SQUIRE, C. VOUT,
T. J. G. WHITMARSH

IMPAIRED CONSCIOUSNESS IN ANCIENT MEDICAL TEXTS

ANDRÉS D. PELAVSKI
Hebrew University of Jerusalem

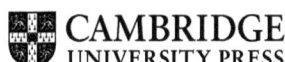
CAMBRIDGE
UNIVERSITY PRESS

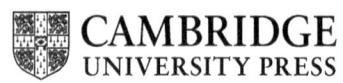

CAMBRIDGE
UNIVERSITY PRESS

Shaftesbury Road, Cambridge CB2 8EA, United Kingdom

One Liberty Plaza, 20th Floor, New York, NY 10006, USA

477 Williamstown Road, Port Melbourne, VIC 3207, Australia

314–321, 3rd Floor, Plot 3, Splendor Forum, Jasola District Centre, New Delhi – 110025, India

103 Penang Road, #05–06/07, Visioncrest Commercial, Singapore 238467

Cambridge University Press is part of Cambridge University Press & Assessment, a department of the University of Cambridge.

We share the University's mission to contribute to society through the pursuit of education, learning and research at the highest international levels of excellence.

www.cambridge.org
Information on this title: www.cambridge.org/9781009616591

DOI: 10.1017/9781009616577

First published 2026

A catalogue record for this publication is available from the British Library

Library of Congress Cataloging-in-Publication Data
NAMES: Pelavski Atlas, Andrés Diego author
TITLE: Impaired consciousness in ancient medical texts / Andrés D. Pelavski.
DESCRIPTION: Cambridge ; New York, NY : Cambridge University Press, 2026. | Series: Cambridge classical studies | Includes bibliographical references and index.
IDENTIFIERS: LCCN 2025015037 | ISBN 9781009616591 hardback | ISBN 9781009616577 ebook | ISBN 9781009616607 paperback
SUBJECTS: LCSH: Loss of consciousness | Altered states of consciousness | Medicine, Ancient
CLASSIFICATION: LCC RB150.L67 P45 2026
LC record available at https://lccn.loc.gov/2025015037

ISBN 978-1-009-61659-1 Hardback
ISBN 978-1-009-61660-7 Paperback

CONTENTS

Contents

PREFACE

This book looks at ancient medical descriptions of patients with disturbed behaviours, altered sleep and swoons (three presentations of what we nowadays designate as impaired consciousness), in order to explore if and how their authors conceived the notion of consciousness. Undoubtedly, such a construct intersects with diverse non-technical discourses (including philosophy, religion, literary and art representations), and medical writers – as individuals immersed in their respective societies – were not alien to them. Nevertheless, my analysis will mainly focus on the scientific debate (with only minor digressions about other areas of thought and culture, whenever they are key to understanding the textual evidence).

The rationale for such a decision is that doctors' subject matter is eminently practical and goal oriented, hence their engagement with extra-medical debates in technical works is often guided by these goals, even when discussing theoretical issues. We can see it very clearly nowadays: no doctor could provide a universally accepted definition of consciousness, yet they are able to diagnose, treat and discuss cases where it is impaired. In antiquity the limits between science and other disciplines were certainly more blurred. However, as we shall see, the authors under discussion tended to orient their reflections towards the practice (that is, towards resolving determined conditions). Even a philosophically informed author such as Galen often used his vast erudition to tweak prestigious thinkers' ideas in support of his own medical explanations, based on his successful cures. Ultimately, even when discussing issues beyond the strictly medical domain, rather than engaging in pure abstract speculation, the goal of most of these writers' reflections and theorisations was to find, to justify or to support a certain therapy.

The scope of this book is, therefore, circumscribed to the 'heuristic role of impaired consciousness'[1] within the medical discourse, namely, this condition will be used to understand the way in which the notion of consciousness was conceived by some doctors who tried to reverse such impairment. I will not tackle representations of the concept outside the medical corpus in depth, nor will I discuss how changing ideas about human action, or the evolving relations between men and gods might have impinged upon these doctors' understanding of consciousness.

In terms of organisation, I propose a dual approach to the material: a longitudinal thematic axis, developed in the course of the three parts in which the book is divided, will illuminate how ideas about impaired consciousness changed and evolved over time. This axis will allow us to contrast continuities and disruptions within each of the three clinical presentations (delirium, sleep and fainting) in the different authors. At all times, in a methodologically self-conscious manner to avoid bias and anachronistic extrapolations, I will make allusions to our current theoretical understanding of these matters.

The transversal axis, on the other hand, follows each group of medical writers (HC, post-Hellenistic authors and Galen) across the different parts of the book, in order to examine issues that are specific for each source (irrespective of their particular take on the main topic under discussion).

---

[1] Devinant (2020: 301).

ACKNOWLEDGEMENTS

This book originated as a doctoral thesis, submitted to the University of Cambridge in 2020. As such, I would like to thank first and foremost my supervisor, Professor Rebecca Flemming. Her insightful challenges and questions help me to approach ancient documents to this day. I feel enormous gratitude for her support, encouragement and warmth throughout that journey and beyond.

Additionally, I feel indebted to Dr. Myrto Hatzimichali and Dr. David Leith for their thorough reading of my research, their useful suggestions, and the stimulating discussion during my viva voce examination.

My appreciation extends further to the Faculty of Classics, who accepted me as a part-time student, partially funded the course, and granted my dissertation the annual Hare Prize. Outside the academic sphere, I want to thank my friend David Rodriguez, who generously contributed to the design of the cover, and I would also like to mention the former and current heads of the Anaesthesia Department of Vall d'Hebron University Hospital, M. Isabel Rochera, Susana Manrique and Anna Gonzalez, who have allowed me a flexible timetable that made (and still makes) it possible to reconcile my clinical duties with my humanistic interests.

Finally, I am thankful to my partner, Paul, for having convinced me to apply to Cambridge in the first place, and for having inspired and cheered me up throughout all these years.

ABBREVIATIONS

Primary sources are cited in the text following the standard abbreviations, as they appear in the *Greek-English Lexicon* by G. Liddell and R. Scott (LSJ, 9th Ed. 1940, Oxford: Clarendon Press). Every passage is referenced with its abbreviated title and the corresponding numeration according to the edition used, which can both be found in the Bibliography section. For the sake of clarity the edition is often also specified within the text.

All the quotations from the Hippocratic and the Galenic corpora are taken from the last available edition. For the abbreviations and English titles I followed Craik (2015) and Singer (2013), respectively. Both editions and abbreviations are detailed in the Bibliography.

Translations from all Greek and Latin sources are my own unless otherwise stated.

ANRW	*Aufstieg und Niedergang der Römischen Welt.*
C	E.M. Craik's edition of the Hippocratic treatise *On glands.*
CMG	*Corpus Medicorum Graecorum.*
CUF	*Collection des Universités Françaises* (Budé edition, *Les belles lettres*).
Ed.	Edition.
Edit.	Editor.
GCS	Glasgow Coma Scale.
G	B. Gundert's edition of Galen's *On the distinction of symptoms.*
H	K. Hude's edition of the works of Aretaeus (from the *CMG*).
HC	Hippocratic corpus.
HOFs	Higher order functions.
K	C.G. Kuhn's edition of the Galenic corpus.
LCL	Loeb Classical Library.

M	J.E. Mann's edition of Hippocratic treatise *The art of medicine.*
Teubner	*Bibliotheca Scriptorum Graecorum et Romanorum Teubneriana.*

Ancient texts are quoted according to the following model (except for Budé edition, where the model is slightly different):

abridged title.	*volume. chapter.*	*modern edition (edit.). volume:*	page, lines;	*reference ed.* (when suitable)
SD I	6.	*CMG (H).III:*	42, 31–2; 43	
MM	*XIII.21.*	*LCL III:*	400, 7–11	*K.X:* 928–9.

Model for the Budé edition:

abridged title.	*modern edition*	*volume.chapter:* case (when suitable), page, lines;	*reference ed.* (when suitable)
Vict.	*CUF*	*4.86:* 2, 12–13	
Ars. Med.	*CUF*	*5.2:* 287, 1–2	*K.I:* 319.

CHAPTER I

INTRODUCTION: MANY DEFINITIONS OF CONSCIOUSNESS

Consciousness means different things to different people,[1] and debates around it exist in many disciplines. What in lay terms is conceived as 'the feeling of being inside oneself looking out' or as 'having a soul' bears testimony to a long tradition that is still nowadays discussed among doctors, neuroscientists and philosophers, to name but a few.[2] Indeed, the topic triggers recurrent polemic about perceptual experiences and bodily sensations, as well as questions regarding mental imagery, emotions, thoughts and behaviours. As a result, it is not unusual that according to the context and the field of research, the notion acquires different nuances, where overlapping ideas such as 'awareness', 'wakefulness', 'sentience' are often involved and not seldom confused.[3]

This book aims to explore some ancient medical contributions to this tradition. To do it, it will analyse a few accounts of impaired consciousness that spread out over a substantial geographical and chronological extension, namely, from Greece, Rome and Asia Minor; and between the Greek classical period (around the fifth century BCE) and the heights of the Roman Empire (in the second century CE). Whilst contextualising the different works amid their contemporary debates, the analysis will explore the scientific milieu in which the texts were conceived, as well as the chronologic changes in medical thought from one period to the other.

Sources

Given the breadth of the chosen temporal frame, and in order to narrow down the scope of the project, I will focus on a limited number of sources. The selection was based on their relevance within medical historiography; their varied approaches to the

---

[1] Rao (1988: 310).   [2] Burkeman (2014).   [3] Carmel and Spreavak (2015: 103–4).

subject, which allow different perspectives; our access to their direct tradition; and the completeness of their extant works, that is, whole texts were preferred because they enable a more comprehensive understanding of the writers' stance. (Hellenistic authors are not dealt with in-depth, because their evidence is mainly doxographic and often fragmentary, thereby entailing a serious risk of deformation and misinterpretation.)[4]

In terms of specific texts, I have divided the authors into three groups: a selection of treatises from the Hippocratic corpus,[5] some post-Hellenistic books (particularly, Celsus' *On medicine*, and *On the causes, symptoms and cure of acute and chronic diseases* by Aretaeus of Cappadocia),[6] and a few works by Galen, the great physician of the Roman Empire.[7]

Hippocratic corpus and Hippocratic authors

From the Hippocratic corpus, I am particularly interested in signalling some general views on impaired consciousness shared by different practitioners, which challenge the often-flagged heterogeneity in terms of genres,[8] origins,[9] voices,[10] theories and perspectives.[11] Indeed, modern researchers struggle to find widespread ideas or

---

[4] The main extant sources for studying this period are some quotations and reports by Rufus and Soranus of Ephesus, the third section of the *Anonymus Londinensis*, Celsus' work and especially, Galen (Longrigg 1993: 182–3).

[5] The particular choice of works – inevitably arbitrary, as any other selection – tries to reflect the wide variety of genres and approaches to impaired consciousness that the collection offers. They are all pre-Aristotelian and I will designate their medical writers collectively as 'Hippocratic authors'.

[6] 'Post-Hellenistic' refers to medical writers from the first and early second century CE (excluding Galen, who will be discussed separately). Their works incorporate and build on crucial scientific developments from the Hellenistic period to which we no longer have direct access. Beyond Aretaeus and Celsus, references will be made to two didactic handbooks wrongly attributed to Galen, the *Introduction* and the *Medical definitions*, as well as the *Anonymus Parisinus*, a catalogue of diseases, where the author summarises the points of view of prestigious doctors.

[7] From Galen's extensive production I have selected nine treatises belonging to different genres, where impaired consciousness is addressed from various perspectives: *On the distinction of diseases* (*Morb. Diff.*), *On the causes of diseases* (*Caus. Morb.*), *On the distinction of symptoms* (*Symp. Diff.*), *On the causes of symptoms* (*Caus. Symp.*), *Coma according to Hippocrates* (*Com. Hipp.*), *The method of medicine* (*MM*), *On the affected parts* (*Loc. Aff.*), *The art of medicine* (*Ars. Med.*) and *The capacities of the soul follow the mixtures of the body* (*QAM*).

[8] Lonie (1983: 148).   [9] Jouanna (2018: 39).   [10] Craik (2018: 29).

[11] Nutton (2013a: 60).

constructs that remain consistent throughout this first comprehensive textual testimony of Greek learned medicine.[12] Scholars tend to limit such coincidences mostly to the period that these practitioners inhabited – characterised by the 'seismic social, cultural, and intellectual changes' that accompanied the emergence of written prose to communicate ideas – and by their stance as a group: they identified themselves and their *technê* by distinction from other disciplines, and developed a form of literary expression to claim authority.[13]

On the contrary, I aim to show that both from a conceptual and a terminological point of view, these authors shared some rudimentary ideas regarding consciousness. In this sense, I will argue that the Hippocratic collection witnesses a 'theory of mind' and a 'technical vocabulary' in the making. I do not agree with Lloyd's opinion that the situation was 'bordering on terminological anarchy';[14] nor with Holmes' view that 'ideas about the *sôma*, the *psuchê* and human nature were "messily" proliferating in the late fifth and early fourth century BCE' (at least in this respect).[15] I shall claim that there was a consistent – though vague and ill-defined – embryonic notion of consciousness, which underlies several Hippocratic accounts, and that doctors were struggling to delimit the concept.

Post-Hellenistic authors

The massive loss of textual evidence from Hellenistic Alexandria[16] and its prominent figures, Herophilus and Erasistratus,[17] makes it difficult for us to explore elusive notions such as consciousness in this period. We can, at best, catch small glimpses of the main sectarian debates regarding Hellenistic developments through our post-Hellenistic medical writers, who quoted, challenged or

---

[12] Actually, we can define this material as 'loosely' medical because along with the discussions about the body and its diseases, there is a wealth of ethnographic, historical and philosophical considerations (Cross, 2018: 4).
[13] Dean-Jones (2003: 102–3).   [14] Lloyd (1983: 163).   [15] Holmes (2010: 32).
[16] Lang (2013: 243–67) offers a good summary of the main features of the medical activity in Alexandria.
[17] Longrigg (1993: 474–5), von Staden (1989) and Garofalo (1988) have published the most complete collection, to date, of the remaining fragments by Herophilus and Erasistratus, respectively.

supported their forerunners.[18] As a result, when analysing this group of sources, particular attention will be paid to the way in which their authors positioned themselves in the face of alternative or rival discourses, as well as their strategies to acquire and organise knowledge. Naturally, all these issues were strongly dependent on the specific period that each writer lived in, on the kind of project that they were carrying out and on the ongoing debates that surrounded each of them.

As will transpire from the discussion, the Hellenistic discoveries of the nervous system and its functioning – especially, their understanding of the body, its movement and perceptions – are of particular importance for later doctors' conceptions of impaired consciousness.

Aulus Cornelius Celsus

On medicine is a paradigmatic example of Roman encyclopaedism, a phenomenon related to a strong quest for learning among the upper classes, paralleled by a substantial expansion in the book-world.[19] As such, its eight volumes provide us with a systematic digest of practical medical knowledge[20] available to the Roman elites during the early Republic.[21]

As with the Hippocratic authors, we are faced with a plurality of voices claiming authority. However, in Celsus' project the alternative discourses have been filtered by a single writer, whose job involved picking out a few texts, ignoring several others and articulating opposing views. Celsus construes the evolution of medicine as a genealogy of disagreements, and positions himself at all times 'somehow in the middle between opposite opinions'.[22] His legitimacy (thus, his claim to authority) relied on demonstrating

---

[18] Nutton (2013a: 135–8). See also von Staden (2002: 83–91).   [19] Contino (2000: 49).

[20] Although his work is theory laden, Celsus avoids theoretical discussions beyond the *prooemium*. As Mudry (2006a: 12) has remarked, not even his descriptions of diseases are exhaustive; he merely outlines some distinctive traits that enable the reader to recognise them, but his focus is on treatment.

[21] Langslow (1994: 300) has defined the audience as 'amateur Roman *curantes*'. Undoubtedly, medical literacy was useful for the *patresfamiliae*, who needed to make relevant medical decisions when choosing doctors for their household, and interacting with them (Flemming, 2000: 59).

[22] *media quodammodo diversas in sententias* (*Med.* I. Proem. 45).

his qualities as a 'virtuoso reader and critic', and on showing off his 'wide erudition and cunning arrangements'.[23] Despite the long list of doctors referred to in the *prooemium*, the canon of writers that he repeatedly quotes are mainly limited to Asclepiades, Erasistratus and Hippocrates.[24] The analysis of his work will argue that his ideas on impaired consciousness are significantly influenced by corpuscular theories such as Ascelpiades' and the Epicureans'.

Aretaeus of Cappadocia

I will consider Aretaeus as a learned physician from the second half of the first century CE and the first half of the second[25] with an evident commitment to reason, who looked for physical causes as a means to explain health and disease. In other words, he will be regarded as a 'non-sectarian author', or a 'physician without further affiliation', who laid claim to Hippocratic authority.[26] The analysis of his ideas on consciousness will show that, whilst his explanations did not strictly fit in any single philosophical system or sect, they laxly referred to several of them.[27]

Although he likely shared with Celsus a profound awareness of the Hellenistic tradition, and both their projects presuppose several voices underpinning an allegedly single discourse, Aretaeus did not feel the need to make alternative opinions compatible. He simply generated knowledge by choosing whichever theory better explained a specific point that he wanted to make, regardless of whether they contradicted (syncretism) or were compatible with (synthesis) other later assertions.[28] Consequently, I will argue that,

---

[23] König and Woolf (2013: 36).   [24] von Staden (1994a: 83).

[25] Oberhelman (1993: 958–9) offers an overview of the centuries-lasting debate regarding Aretaeus' chronology and sectarian belonging. He limits his *floruit* to the latter part of the first century CE, whereas Perez Molina (1998: 14) is less categorical and widens the bracket. I agree with the latter, for Oberhelman's argument is based on ascribing Aretaeus to a certain sect, which I will challenge.

[26] Flemming (2012: 70, 79).

[27] Whereas Wellmann considered him as an Eclectic, Oberhelman (1993: 958) and Stannard (1964: 30) highlight the Stoic basis of his Pneumatic approach. Other authors nuance these views: McDonald (2009b: 118) sees in his work the Hippocratic influence on Pneumatic medicine, and Pigeaud (1987: 85) acknowledges the role of *pneuma* in Aretaeus' theory, but questions whether he can be exclusively ascribed to the Pneumatic school.

[28] Syncretism supposes an uncritical juxtaposition of ideas that fails to reconcile heterodox views (Albrecht, 1994: 104); synthesis is the opposite phenomenon, that is, when

5

based on his understanding of impaired consciousness, it makes sense to characterise his approach as eclectic,[29] even while avoiding any implication in terms of his belonging to the Eclectic sect (if such a group ever existed).

In other words, my reading of his work will suggest that he embraced eclecticism as an 'intellectual attitude',[30] and I shall describe it as 'lax' eclecticism to distinguish it from the Eclectic sect. In his use of the terminology and his appropriation of others' ideas we can, at best, find a certain 'family resemblance' with different well-known theoretical frameworks available during his lifetime, but he does not fully commit to any of them.[31]

Galen of Pergamum

As opposed to the abundant philosophical scholarly research on Galen's psychology, this analysis will look at his understanding of impaired consciousness from the more medical side of the debate. My argument aims to show how Galen's take on impaired consciousness is based on the intersection of two theoretical traditions: the anatomical and the humoural, both of which were part of the intellectual zeitgeist.[32]

---

diverse ideas are successfully combined, without evident contradiction amongst them (Donini, 1988: 21). *Sumphorêsis* – from '*sumpephorêmenos*' (mixed, jumbled) – is a coinage inspired by Epicurus' criticism of philosophers who disregard the semantic distinctions for the same term across different philosophical systems (Hatzimichali, 2011: 19). All three concepts have been associated with eclecticism.

[29] Eclecticism has been defined as 'an intellectual stance that involves approving of and adopting views that are not part of a uniform tradition, but might stem from different, even incompatible, ideologies' (Hatzimichali, 2011: 9).

[30] In his analysis of eclecticism in modern philosophy, Schneider (1998: 177) draws a useful distinction between doctrinal eclecticism as opposed to an eclectic 'intellectual attitude'.

[31] Wittgenstein's account of family resemblance is useful for characterising Aretaeus' approach. The idea that a general concept (in this case a general theory) applies to all the particular instances (in the explanations) by virtue of some specific feature or principle that is shared by all such explanations does not apply in Aretaeus' examples. On the contrary, we find that theories apply by virtue of multiple features or principles only shared by certain subsets of such explanations in a criss-crossing and overlapping manner (Forster 2010: 67). Consequently, instead of a single theory (or sect, or school of thought) that captures and underpins all Aretaeus' work, we are faced with a network of concepts that belong to different theories, which are constantly crossing and intersecting.

[32] I disagree with Pigeaud's idea that there is a breach between 'fine anatomy' and 'humouralism, which guides therapeutics' (2008: 582). On the contrary, I will claim

On the one hand, the anatomical expertise, which Galen had gained through dissection with the most prestigious teachers,[33] provided him with the *locus affectus*, namely, the bodily location where the compromise occurred, hence, where treatments needed to be aimed at.[34] On the other, Galen drew his pathophysiological explanations from the theory of the four humours (*chumoi*). His merit was to articulate these allegedly Hippocratic ideas with the theory of the four elements (*stoicheia*) – which after Empedocles had exerted a powerful influence on philosophical thought.[35] The nexus that enabled him to bridge elements with humours was the notion of qualities (*poiotêtes*), which had been independently related to both systems for centuries.[36] As Schöner pointed out, although only one step was missing to join both theories, 500 years went by before Galen established such a relationship.[37]

The hot, the cold, the dry and the wet underpinned the theory of mixtures (*kraseis*), whereby diseases were caused by an imbalance of qualities (*duskrasia*).[38] Through this move, Galen was able to claim the prestige of both the philosophical elemental tradition and the Hippocratic humoural one, while he actually moved away from both towards a system based mainly on qualities. Furthermore, this approach offered Galen a qualitative and quantitative framework to guide the choice of allopathic therapies. In his system the kind of

that both are constantly in play, and that it is their precise combination which determines the type and site of the therapy required.

[33] Gourevitch and Grmek (1994: 1493–525) offer a thorough account of Galen's educational journeys.

[34] According to McDonald (2011: 63, 76), this concept had emerged in the post-classical period and achieved its fullest expression with Galen. Although Archigenes had shown a keen interest in the topic, he based his treatments on an authoritative therapeutic tradition, but not on the physiological theories that he supported (Lewis, 2018: 172). It was Galen who took the crucial step of integrating anatomy and humoural pathophysiology into diagnosis and treatment.

[35] Very schematically, Galen considered that the primary elements (water, fire, air, and earth) were formed out of matter and qualities (*hulês* and *poiotêtôn*). The former, in turn, constituted the whole cosmos, and entered the body through food and drink, in order to compose the humours (blood, phlegm, yellow and black bile). The latter, finally, constituted the homogeneous parts that were components of the organs (*Hip. Elem. CMG VIII*: 126, 5–9 –K. I. 479, 480).

[36] Already in *On the nature of man* (fourth century BCE) each humour was related to a couple of qualities and a time of the year (*De Nat. Hom. CMG VII*: 182–6). Similarly, Plato (*Tim.* 82A–B) related the imbalance of elements and qualities to diseases, and Aristotle (*P.A. II.1*: 646a 13–24) attributed certain qualities to each element.

[37] Schöner (1964: 65).   [38] Jouanna (2012: 339).

7

duskrasia was crucial not only to determine the type of qualities imbalanced – which needed to be opposed – but also the degree of their disturbance. Thus, the skilled doctor was able to choose the drug that would have the exact potency to counterbalance the level of disturbance of each altered quality within the mixture.

In summary, with these three components – bodily location, quality disturbed and degree of disturbance – Galen developed a coherent, cohesive and efficient system to address possible disturbances of consciousness. We shall see that whenever such conditions were under discussion Galen funnelled the arguments into this tripartite scheme, which could be effectively managed by his medicine, thereby providing him with authority.[39]

Definitions of consciousness: perspectives, specificity and pitfalls

An initial hurdle for the present undertaking – exploring impaired consciousness in these authors – is the vagueness of its key concept. Scholars grapple with definitions of consciousness because they vary substantially across different theoretical frameworks. This possibly enriches the debate by illuminating alternative perspectives, but also leaves it rather unresolved. Below are a few examples of attempts at systematising this elusive notion.

Broadly speaking, philosophers of mind have distinguished between two types of constructs: an easily accessible one, which according to Block involves the rational control of thought and action, and therefore is designated as 'access consciousness', and the more elusive 'phenomenal consciousness'.[40] While the former is objective, representational and comprised of verbally transmittable contents, such as thoughts, desires and beliefs,[41] the latter refers to the subjective feelings that accompany mental processes. Phenomenal consciousness comprises the 'qualia' or subjective

[39] As von Staden has remarked (1997: 36), Galen's claim to authority was influenced by the values of the Second Sophistic. Within his self-construed image as a *pepaideumenos* physician, his system – legitimised by the alleged endorsement of the ancients, his outspoken studies in philosophy and logic, and his own experience – is used as a powerful argument to discredit rivals and promote himself.

[40] Block (2002: 207).   [41] Carmel and Spreavak (2015: 104).

experiences that respond to the question 'what is it like?' In this sense, 'an organism is conscious if there is something it is like to be that organism'.[42] Why and how that 'inner life' – that is, phenomenal consciousness – arises is, according to Chalmers, the hard problem.[43]

On the other hand, neuroscientists have mainly attempted to tackle the allegedly 'easy' problems, namely, the neural correlates of consciousness. In general terms, they have focused on understanding the patterns of brain activity that determine different levels of consciousness, and the processes that shape our perceptual awareness.[44] In this manner, they have isolated different components such as 'wakefulness' or level of consciousness, and 'awareness', which refers to the content thereof. This concept can be further subdivided into external (awareness of our surrounding environment) and internal (our inner world). Thus, by combination of these independent components neuroscientists classify various possible states of consciousness.[45]

Because doctors are forced to work at the practical interface between the mental (including the phenomenal) and the bodily (including the neurophysiological) aspects of consciousness,[46] they have been more successful in describing and assessing its impairment, rather than actually defining it in itself. Even if the concept as such is not unequivocally delimited, conditions with altered levels of consciousness are quite common, well-characterised and quantifiable clinical findings. Indeed, they are ubiquitous and easily recognisable in current medical practice: not only in physiological processes, such as spontaneous sleep, but also induced by certain substances such as anaesthetics or recreational drugs. Furthermore, they are common during various types of disease, both mental and physical.

In everyday practice, changes in consciousness are considered to belong in a continuous spectrum that ranges from patients who are 'awake, alert and appropriate' (that is, normally functioning individuals) to deep coma and vegetative states. Between these extremes, several levels of drowsiness, agitation, delirium and

---

[42] Nagel (1974: 435–50).   [43] Chalmers (2010: 5).
[44] Carmel and Spreavak (2015: 109).   [45] Laureys (2007: 32–7).
[46] Fulford (2006: 24–5).

confusion have been singled out. As will be shown below, ever since antiquity, physicians have strived to measure, grade and label these various states of consciousness and have devised tools to achieve this goal. The famous Glasgow Coma Scale (GCS) – created around the mid-1970s[47] – is a relatively recent example to numerically quantify the level of consciousness. As will be discussed, other arguably similar attempts (which even utilise surprisingly similar parameters) date back to as early as the Hippocratic corpus.

In other words, this book aims to identify in ancient texts an extremely common medical finding that stands at the interface between physiological and pathological phenomena, and between what we consider as 'mental' and 'somatic' conditions. Inevitably, the way in which ancient doctors framed such situations was influenced by other deeper understandings about the workings of the soul, the mind and the body, which the analysis will try to expose.

Working definition of consciousness

It is evident from the above – even after this short glimpse at only three disciplines – that each specialist (whether philosopher, doctor or neurobiologist) approaches the matter in a particular way, asks specific questions and fragments consciousness into distinct components according to those questions. The picture would become even more intricate if we dug deeper into any of these fields of study, let alone if we added other areas of knowledge where consciousness was also addressed. As a result, it looks as though this concept precluded any attempt at a universal, comprehensive, clear-cut definition. Such Aristotle-inspired lists of essential criteria and attributes seem inadequate for these kinds of complex notions, which acquire different nuances depending on the aspect being addressed, and whose boundaries are often 'fuzzy'.[48]

Alternatively, in order to establish what I will regard as belonging within the sphere of consciousness and its impairment, I have used a cognitive model inspired by Rosch.[49] Beyond the evident

---

[47] Teasdale and Jennet (1974: 81–4).   [48] Aitchinson (1994).   [49] Rosch (1975).

advantage of bypassing the impossibility of establishing strict boundaries to such an elusive construct, this approach has the added benefit of allowing an analysis of compatible ideas on consciousness – in antiquity and nowadays – without anachronistic assumptions.

According to this model, classifying objects into a category requires establishing relationships between those objects and an ideal exemplar that represents the most typical case within that category, or its 'prototype'. In this way, each member within a group shares only certain characteristics with the prototype (not all of them, and different members share different characteristics with it).[50] Additionally, by matching the features of a certain object to an ideal exemplar, one can determine the extent to which that object identifies with the prototype, and hence, how much it belongs to the category. This introduces another advantage to this model, which is the membership gradience, namely, the idea that different members have different degrees of affiliation to a category.[51] As a result, this model is also capable of reflecting the above-mentioned tendency among doctors of all eras to distinguish different levels of consciousness: ultimately, the closer a condition resembles a prototype that defines impaired consciousness, the lower the level of consciousness of that condition.

In our current medical understanding there are three easily recognisable clinical presentations that we nowadays unequivocally consider within the compromised end of the spectrum of consciousness. They are delirium (or wakeful impaired consciousness), sleep (or drowsy impaired consciousness) and fainting (or total loss of consciousness). I shall use them as prototypes to identify the phenomenon in antiquity. They will function in the discussion as ideal exemplars; namely, I will assume that the medical writers were talking about impaired consciousness whenever their accounts resembled one of these three presentations. To avoid the trap of importing anachronistic concepts into the texts,[52]

---

[50] Aitchinson (1994) explains the usefulness of this model to categorise what he defines as words with 'fuzzy edges', that is, words whose limits are uncertain. Given that consciousness has very 'fuzzy edges', the prototype model seems like a valid method to approach the definition challenges.
[51] Lackoff (1987: 13).   [52] Singer (1992: 132).

I will not presuppose that ancient doctors actually had an idea of consciousness. On the contrary, I shall simply explore how they framed – and how (if at all) they linked in their discourse – certain conditions, in which their patients suffered swoons, slept too much or too little, talked nonsense or were simply not their usual selves. Ultimately, my aim is to understand what they made of these findings (which they often described and acknowledged within their sphere of expertise, and which we nowadays regard as paradigmatic examples of impaired consciousness); how they related them to other ideas and beliefs; and to assess the extent to which they perceived them as connected conditions. By doing so I aim to single out this concept, generally overlooked by scholars, which reflects a distinct reality and permeates different aspects of these doctors' more general beliefs, including ideas about the soul, the body, illness and even death. . .

Similarities and contrasts between the three prototypes of impaired consciousness

There is a further set of subcategories (in a lower hierarchical level) that will be useful in thinking about the relationships among these three prototypical presentations. As a matter of fact, much like the idea of consciousness itself, delirium, sleep and fainting also present fuzzy edges between them, and there are certain situations where it is difficult to separate one from another (this is why we nowadays consider impaired consciousness as a continuous spectrum and not as a collection of discrete independent states). For instance, vivid nightmares with sleepwalking can be hard to distinguish from wakeful delirious states with hallucinations. Similarly, it is not always straightforward to differentiate cases of fainting from episodes of deep dreamless sleep. To overcome this hurdle and articulate such ambiguous interphases between prototypical presentations, there is a network of concepts that provides a simple theoretical framework. It is comprised of three notions: 'alertness', 'connectedness' and 'responsiveness'.

Anaesthetists, whose job is to manage and regulate different levels of consciousness, explain physiological and pathological states through these notions, as well as the above-mentioned shifts and the grey areas between them. Alertness is the ability to experience and perform intellectual tasks, to reason, to plan, to acknowledge perceptions, and the awareness of these functions as belonging to the self. Connectedness alludes to our link with the inner and outer world, that is, internal and environmental connections which enable us to experience stimuli. Finally, responsiveness refers to our complex behavioural interactions with our surroundings. It can be spontaneous or goal-directed (when obeying an order).[53]

Different combinations of these concepts can explain both undisturbed and altered levels of consciousness. In the normal wakeful state, individuals are typically alert, connected and responsive. Similarly, in dreams – which are normal physiological states – alertness is intact (we can perceive and perform intellectual operations during oneiric experiences), but there is a lack of connectedness to the environment and no responsiveness. Conversely, in dreamless sleep all three are absent. On the other hand, abnormal states – such as delirium – can be characterised by various combinations of malfunctioning. In some cases connection to the environment is intact (perception is preserved) but alertness fails. Such patients can normally receive environmental stimuli but are incapable of complex processing; in other words, their cognition is impaired. The degree of responsiveness in these cases will determine whether we talk of hyperactive impaired consciousness, where the patient moves, resists, acts aggressively or speaks incomprehensibly, or hypoactive impaired consciousness such as drowsy states or 'coma vigil' (in which the affected individual can open their eyes, but is otherwise completely unconscious with no response whatsoever).

These concepts are particularly useful in understanding the fuzzy edges, namely, the links and interfaces where the boundaries between these prototypes become blurred. In this sense, the similarities between vivid dreams and delirium can be framed as conditions with preserved alertness and impaired connectedness to the environment, for both are present in nightmares and wakeful hallucinations. Similarly, the difficulty of distinguishing between swoons and deep dreamless sleep can be explained by

---

the coincidence in the complete abolition of alertness, connectedness and responsiveness that occurs in both. In other words, the advantage of dividing the prototypical presentations into these subcategories is that they highlight the grey areas where they touch each other and help us understand the points where syndromes can be easily confused. This model will be particularly useful in grasping the reality underlying some ancient medical sources.

A brief glance at recent scholarship

There has been growing interest in mental disorders in antiquity during the last few decades, as evidenced by the interdisciplinary approaches from which they have been tackled. However, scholars have persistently avoided discussing consciousness.[54] Due to the nature of the ancient descriptions, they have, instead, funnelled these accounts into two main thematic discussions. They have either framed them as cases of madness (failing to distinguish between delirium and mental illness) or as evidence of ancient philosophical debates on psychology.[55] Regardless of whether the focus of discussion is limited to a particular author, a specific aspect or a more general analysis of the topic across different ancient sources, the approaches tend to lean towards one of these two groups.

The model that addresses madness – perhaps influenced by current controversies in the domain of mental health – usually yields psychiatrically informed analyses that attempt to fit descriptions found in ancient texts into contemporary classifications of mental illness.[56] However, such an exercise demonstrates our own

---

[54] Harris' book (2013) on mental disorders offers a good example, for he presents a collection of studies from rich and diverse perspectives, but there is no allusion whatsoever to impaired consciousness.

[55] From the first group the main representative bibliography is: Pigeaud (1987), Pigeaud (1994), Stok (1996), Murphy (2013), Nutton (2013b), McDonald (2014). From the second: van der Eijk (2005), Tieleman (2003). Naturally, there are several other analyses (which will be discussed in the different chapters), where scholars lean towards one of these approaches. The above-mentioned ones are just a sample of the most relevant.

[56] Benett (2013: 27–40), and Hugues (2013: 41–58) both draw parallels between the *Diagnostic and Statistic Manual* (DSM) of the American Psychiatric Association and some ancient classification endeavours. Possibly the most radical example within this

difficulty in categorising mental disease, rather than exploring the ancients' view on these matters. Moreover, in most of these studies there is a caveat with the construct 'mental illness'. It is either conceived differently by each scholar, depending on the aspect that they are trying to highlight, or the concept is so broadly and vaguely defined that it ends up being inadequate to distinguish specific conditions, such as impaired consciousness.[57]

Regarding the approach that looks at the philosophical reading of these passages, modern scholarship tends to explore notions such as mind, soul and their anatomical location.[58] Under the overarching construct of the mind, authors have made inquiries into the functioning and interaction of body, thought, spirit and intelligence,[59] as well as into theories about the substances involved.[60] Even if scattered allusions to consciousness might arise in such discussions,[61] authors seldom remark on some links that the ancients intuited between unusual perceptions, sleep disturbances and behaviours perceived as abnormal. In general, most approaches to these texts have discussed the peripheries – or the fuzzy edges – of impaired consciousness, but they have not been able to reach to its core.

Grmek is one of the few exceptions, for he posited that most Hippocratic descriptions were not referring to psychotic disorders,

group is Matentzoglu's thesis (Matentzoglu 2011: 16–18), where she looks for 'psycho-pathological symptoms' in the Hippocratic descriptions, and utilises the *International Classification of Diseases* (ICD-10) to provide a systematic phenomenological classification of them. Also within this group, Devinant (2020) grapples with delimiting the 'psychic troubles' in the Galenic corpus.

57 A good example of the latter problem is the recent book by C. Thumiger (2017), which offers a very interesting analysis of these issues. However, by defining her object of study as a 'continuum between pathology and sanity' (46), and considering 'every mental sign as a manifestation of madness' (44), she eliminates any possibility of more specific or nuanced characterisations.

58 Hankinson (1991: 194–217).

59 Gundert (2000: 13–35). Bartos (2015: 185–222) and Devinant (2020) have touched upon the relationship between body and soul in the Hippocratic *On regimen* and in the Galenic corpus, respectively.

60 van der Eijk (2005: 119–35).

61 Gundert (2000: 18) mentions the temporary loss of consciousness in the Hippocratic corpus and van der Eijk (2005: 127) translates *phronêsis* as consciousness (as opposed to *sunesis*). Pigeaud (1987: 14–21) even acknowledges that the ancient texts are not discussing psychopathological conditions, but the loss and recovery of lucidity, which he relates to the field of consciousness. Nevertheless, he explicitly disregards this aspect and focuses on '*la folie*' (1987: 15).

but to *'obnubilations de la conscience'*. Unfortunately, he did not pursue this hypothesis further.[62] In a similar manner, Boehm's analysis of 'unconsciousness and insensitivity in the Hippocratic collection' suggests an association between sensory perceptions and the spirit (*l'esprit*), thereby identifying their impairment with a state of unconsciousness.[63] Nevertheless, despite the title, her study is more focused on insensitivity than on unconsciousness, which, again, is barely tackled. Padel, on the other hand, does embark upon an original scrutiny of the manifestations and representations of consciousness in Athenian tragedy. Although not specifically medical, her thorough study draws some interesting conclusions about the Hippocratic corpus, which will be useful to contrast with the rest of our sources.[64]

Because the idea of impaired consciousness challenges most of the recent scholarly theorisations, the present analysis will primarily attempt to revisit – with this novel framework – the usual set of questions concerning the mind, the soul, the body and their workings. In this way I aim to provide fresh perspectives on these older debates. At all times, my goal will be to ascertain if and how different authors – belonging to diverse traditions and historical periods – perceived the notion of consciousness. These understandings will shed light on their authors' ideas about human functioning more generally, as well as how they conceived the relationship between mind–body–soul, health–disease and life–death.

---

[62] Grmek (1983: 412).   [63] Boehm (2002: 257–70).   [64] Padel (1994).

PART I

DELIRIUM

DEFINITIONS OF DELIRIUM/WAKEFUL IMPAIRED CONSCIOUSNESS VERSUS MADNESS, AND THE CONCEPT OF 'DISEASE'

Among the three prototypical clinical presentations within the spectrum of consciousness, delirium (that is, wakeful impaired consciousness) is undoubtedly the most controversial. Unlike sleep and fainting, which the ancients presumably designated in a similar manner as we currently do, this condition has been less clearly defined and has always prompted more theoretical elaboration. Its changeable nature and ubiquity make the characterisation of delirium less stable, especially considering that it appears in multiple forms and can be present in (and caused by) many other mental or physical, acute or chronic conditions.[1]

First and foremost, it should be emphasised that delirium is nowadays regarded as a cluster of symptoms rather than a disease[2] in its own right. In other words, we should not confuse the features of wakeful impaired consciousness with some specific underlying diseases that often trigger it (currently included within the psychiatric domain). It is in this regard that I will challenge several classicists' simplistic solution of equating all descriptions of diseases involving cognitive compromise with mental illness. Far from attempting an extrapolation of modern categories into ancient texts, by addressing our current framing of these conditions I aim to make the reader aware of the bias with which we approach the sources. Even assuming the low likelihood of finding equivalences between contemporary and ancient theorisations, it is worth bearing in mind that nowadays mental illness and delirium describe utterly different medical realities. (I shall later discuss how this shift in understanding is not a mere change of names, but enables novel insights into

---

[1] Mental illness, madness and insanity will be used as interchangeable terms, and will be distinguished from wakeful impaired consciousness and delirium (which will also be considered as synonyms).
[2] Disease, illness and infirmity will be used interchangeably.

terminological and philosophical issues crucial to ancient medical – and also legal[3] – thought.)

Current medical understanding and definitions

Our current construction of consciousness as a spectrum has already been mentioned in Chapter 1. It is the intermediate areas of this spectrum, particularly those where patients are awake and hyper- or hypoactive but unaware of or disengaged from their surroundings that can be easily confused with madness. It is, therefore, at these points that definitions need to distinguish these different kinds of affections.

My understanding of delirium/wakeful impaired consciousness follows the DSM 5, where it is defined as an acute and fluctuating syndrome characterised by inattention, disturbed awareness and cognition, and in more serious cases, sleep disturbances and hallucinations.[4] Delirium tends to be episodic, self-limited and changeable.

Mental illness, madness or insanity, on the other hand, are considered as an heterogeneous group of chronic conditions (that is, extended in time), which can present various clinical signs, including extreme moods, hallucinations, delusions, thought disorders and negative symptoms (such as apathy, inexpressiveness and lack of motivation).[5] Only the episodes of 'acute psychosis' – which sometimes occur in the course of these longer processes – can be equated with delirium, and hence considered as a specific form of impaired consciousness. Acutely psychotic patients seem out of touch with reality, confused, and any of the above-mentioned symptoms can be present.

---

[3] The legal implications of distinguishing impaired consciousness from mental illness are discussed elsewhere (Pelavski 2023: 399–426).

[4] These are the components of the definition of delirium in the DSM 5: http://www.gpnotebook.co.uk/simplepage.cfm?ID=x20180624174826437326 (last accessed 8 October 2019).

[5] Cooke (2015: 10–11). It should be emphasised that hallucinations (that is, abnormal sensory perceptions) and delusions, which consist of holding elaborate and complex beliefs, tend to be stereotypical and rather stable in mental illness. Patients often report hearing voices, seeing unusual things or having persecution, conspiratorial or mystical delusions that remain more or less unchanged in time. In cases of delirium this consistency is lacking.

It cannot be emphasised enough that delirium is neither equivalent nor specific to psychiatric disorders and can occur in many other conditions. Actually, more often than not it happens in the context of severe systemic diseases (infections, head trauma, intoxication, burns) and several neurological conditions. In other words, an episode of delirium can be a symptom of madness, but it is much more often a manifestation of other conditions, and – more importantly – mental illness cannot be diagnosed only through a single episode of delirium.

Another condition that compromises 'the mind' in a related and easily mistakable manner is dementia. Patients suffering from dementia are predominantly elderly, and their main characteristic is a chronic and progressive deterioration of the neurocognitive abilities, which interferes with their activities of daily living. Memory, language, visual-spatial skills, judgement and problem-solving capacities tend to be compromised. Serious cases can present depression, apathy, hallucinations, delusions, agitation, insomnia or sleep disturbances. In other words, dementia can also present specific episodes of impaired consciousness in certain moments during its prolonged course.

It seems quite evident from the above that the common feature shared by all these disorders, which sometimes makes differential diagnosis difficult, is the compromising – in one way or another – of the so-called higher order functions (HOFs). This notion subsumes numerous brain capacities including memory, verbal communication, perception, attention (which together allow judgement, decision-making and planning), as well as the bodily manifestation of the former; namely, behaviours, which are the ways in which human beings conduct themselves under certain stimuli, in determined situations or circumstances.[6]

Invariably, delirium, mental illness and dementia affect one or several of these HOFs, hence (to use Aitchinson's terms) their fuzzy edges, which have caused confusion between them, since antiquity up to the present day. As we shall see below, the Hippocratic doctors also had an intuition of these constructs, but contrary to what is implied in recent scholarship, they mostly commented on the compromise of HOFs in acute, changeable

---

[6] Tranel (2003: 621).

and short-lived situations, which we can easily identify as delirium or wakeful impaired consciousness. The later authors that we will analyse, conversely, did pay attention to more persistent and stereotyped disturbances of these HOFs. Nevertheless, they made important efforts to distinguish those chronic conditions from sudden episodic disorders and strived to recognise both types in order to provide a specific treatment for each of them.

Delirium as evidence of changing ideas about disease

Like several other concepts that we have been discussing, a distinct and universally accepted definition of disease can also be problematic, particularly because it acquires different nuances in different specialties. Nevertheless, any modern textbook that addresses medical conditions is, roughly speaking, divided into (at least) four main sections that shape our current idea of illness: clinical presentation, bodily location, aetiology – often related to abnormal functioning, damaged mechanisms or structures – and treatment. It is precisely from the interaction of these elements that the notion of illness or disease emerges. Our construct of any such distinct nosological entity presupposes a unity underlying all these components. Namely, doctors are always – explicitly or implicitly – searching for a cause that alters a certain physiological mechanism in the body, which triggers determined symptoms and which needs to be reverted through certain therapeutic measures to achieve a cure. On the contrary, when that unity fails to exist (or science has not yet discovered a logical explanation to link symptoms, organs, mechanisms and treatment), practitioners talk of syndromes, which are conceived as mere groups of signs and symptoms but not as diseases in their own right.

In order to illuminate the ancient writers' understanding of the construct 'disease', the analysis will be scrutinising the extent to which they organised such elements into a coherent whole. In other words, by looking at the way in which ancient doctors articulated signs and symptoms with the affected parts of the body, the pathophysiological mechanisms and their therapeutic approaches, we will be able to gauge how the concept of disease changed in the medical discourse.

CHAPTER 3

DELIRIUM VERSUS MADNESS AND THE NOTION OF DISEASE IN THE HIPPOCRATIC CORPUS

Impaired consciousness in the Hippocratic corpus: delirium case studies

Over half a millennium separates the literary emergence of Hippocratic medicine from the authors – such as Rufus of Ephesus and Aretaeus the Cappadocian – who usually play starring roles in scholarship on 'mental disorders' in antiquity. Similarly, the appearance of affections such as *mania* or *melancholia*[1] is a product of Hellenistic medical developments. In contrast, Hippocratic texts generally include forms of mental derangement and disturbance – delirium, coma, incoherent speech, hallucinations – as symptoms within a larger array of signs, but there are very few allusions to mental derangement as affections in themselves. This pattern reflects a general Hippocratic looseness in the notion of disease, a preference for listing signs rather than providing abstract definitions. These circumstances notwithstanding, scholars have tended to take these notes about episodes of delirium as proof of a larger category of madness underlying these glimpses, thereby drawing generalising conclusions about ancient psychology and body–mind relationships.

As we shall see below, even if the distinction between chronic mental diseases, on the one hand, and acute and changeable episodes of delirium, on the other, can be found in the corpus, the bulk of cases fall into the latter category. Let us examine three groups of disorders or case studies: two forms of delirium affecting young girls, two cases of alcohol-associated delirium and several discussions about *phrenitis*.

---

[1] I have italicised the medical terms that are still in use in order to avoid suggesting an equivalence of meaning between antiquity and the present.

Delirium versus madness

Delirium in young girls

One of the detailed case histories in *Epidemics III* relates to the daughter of Euryanax: 'A fever seized her' and:

... περὶ δὲ δεκάτην μετὰ τὸν ἱδρῶτα τὸν γενόμενον παρέκρουσε καὶ πάλιν ταχὺ κατενόει ... διαλιποῦσα δὲ δωδεκάτῃ πάλιν πολλὰ παρελήρει ... ἀφ'ἧς δὲ παρέκρουσε τὸ ὕστερον ἀπέθανε ἑβδόμη ... ἀπόσιτος πάντων παρὰ πάντα τὸν χρόνον οὐδ'ἐπεθύμησεν οὐδενός. ἄδιψος οὐδ'ἔπινεν οὐδὲν ἄξιον λόγου. σιγῶσα, οὐδὲν διελέγετο. *Epid. III. CUF I.6*: Case 6–b6: 72, 2; 4; 7; 11–13.

... On the tenth day, after sweating, she was delirious (*parekrouse*) and was soon again rational ... after a brief interlude, on the twelfth day, she became very delirious (*parelêrei*) again ... She died on the seventh day after the last delirium (*parekrouse*). She had an aversion for all food during the whole period, and she desired nothing. Not thirsty, she did not drink anything worth mentioning. She remained silent, did not speak at all.

The author seems to be describing a condition that causes intermittent attacks of impaired consciousness, by introducing certain 'delirium terms' such as *parakrouô* (*krouô* means 'hit' or 'strike') and *paralêreô* (*lêreô* means 'speaking nonsense').[2] First this girl *parekrouse*, then *palin katenoei* and then *palin parelêrei*. The first *palin* points towards an opposition between *parekrouse* and *katenoei*, assuming that her consciousness was initially intact, whereas the second *palin* suggests the equivalence between *parekrouse* and *parelêrei*. Moreover, the identity between the latter pair of verbs is further reinforced by the relative clause that places the death on the seventh day after the last delirium (*aph' ês ... parekrouse to husteron*). It is implied, thereby, that the two episodes – namely the first one, where the girl *parekrouse*, and the second one, where she *parelêrei* – were similar, and the terms, therefore, were interchangeable.[3] (This is the reason why I used 'delirium' and its derivatives as a general term to translate different words.)

Towards the end of the passage, the author recaps the main features of the process and further defines the nature of the

---

[2] I shall claim in Part II of this book, in disagreement with Thumiger (2013: 71–5), that these verbs, as well as *parakoptô* (which also conveys the idea of striking), and others, acquire their meaning not from their etymological roots, but by combining with other terms within the so-called 'phrasal terms'.

[3] The relevance of these terms, which – as we will see – are used as partial synonyms is discussed in the second part of the book.

24

disorder: throughout the whole time, the girl presented hypoactive responsiveness. That is why she neither ate, nor drank, nor desired anything, and most importantly, did not say a word. In terms of the course of the disease, the whole thing lasted nineteen days altogether, which – added to the episodic nature of the attacks – seems to point towards an acute disease with delirious fits, rather than a psychiatric condition.

Although probably referring to a different and longer infirmity, the short treatise *On diseases of girls* addresses the general age-group into which the daughter of Eurianax – also a *parthenos* – falls, and seems to contrast mental illness with episodes of impaired consciousness. The condition described is one that can develop if girls reach marriageable age but are not married. They are then affected by ongoing mental problems within which sudden episodes of delirium or, arguably, acute psychosis can trigger suicidal behaviours in the affected young women. Based on its chronic course and regular pattern, we could label this disease as one of the rare examples of mental illness (according to our current understanding) in the Hippocratic corpus. However, the author also describes acute episodes within this longer-lasting process, where consciousness seems impaired. The account begins with a reflection upon the nature of diseases in general, and the charac-terisation of a group of affections in particular. Eventually, the author focuses on the topic of his core discussion:

... περὶ τῶν δειμάτων, ὁκόσα φοβεῦνται ἰσχυρῶς ἄνθρωποι, ὥστε παραφρονέειν καὶ ὁρῆν δοκέειν δαίμονάς τινας ἐφ᾽ ἑωυτῶν δυσμενέας ... ἔπειτα ἀπὸ τῆς τοιαύτης ὄψιος πολλοὶ ἤδη ἀπηγχονίσθησαν... *Virg. CUF I.1*: 188, 5–10.

... about the terrors, which make people particularly afraid, to the degree that they become delirious (*paraphroneein*) and they think that they can see spirits hostile to them ... Then, as a result of such visions, many end up strangling themselves.

The text expands on this latter condition, and the author appears to be describing a basal state of anxiety and fear (a common accom-panying symptom in psychosis) with crescendos where hallucin-ations take place (*hôste paraphroneein*), which can be potentially mortal because they may lead to self-harm. It is during such acute episodes that consciousness becomes temporarily altered.

25

After this general outline of the course of the disease, the author explains the mechanism of these sudden attacks. Blood is collecting in the womb. It should run out as menstruation begins, but the mouth of the womb does not open, and so more and more blood builds up, with nowhere to go except upwards to the heart and the diaphragm:

ὁκόταν οὖν ταῦτα πληρωθέωσιν ἐμωρώθη ἥ καρδίη, εἶτ᾽ ἐκ τῆς μωρώσιος νάρκη, εἶτ᾽ ἐκ τῆς νάρκης παράνοια ἔλαβεν . . . ἐκ δὲ τῆς καρδίης καὶ τῶν φρενῶν βραδέως παλιρροεῖ – ἐπικάρσιαι γὰρ αἱ φλέβες – καὶ ὁ τόπος ἐπίκαιρος ἔς τε παραφροσύνην καὶ μανίην. . . *Virg. 2.2*: 189, 9–11, 19–22.

When they [the heart and the diaphragm] are full, the heart becomes sluggish. Next, from the sluggishness it grows numb, and then, from the numbness, delirium (*paranoia*) affects [the young girls] . . . From the heart and the diaphragm [the blood] flows back slowly, as the veins are twisted. The site is critical for delirium (*paraphrosunên*) and raging (*maniên*).

The passage seems to confirm the idea of sudden fits within a longer-lasting process, thereby reinforcing our hypothesis of impaired consciousness. Through it, the author is offering a pathophysiological explanation as to why these acute episodes that happen within the chronic condition subside so slowly. Namely, due to the anatomical conformation of the vessels.

Undoubtedly, much more can be extracted from these passages. Suffice to say here that these cases of delirium that affect young girls illustrate the short-lived and changeable nature of the episodes of impaired consciousness (as opposed to the longer and more stereo-typed characteristics of the disease that affects unmarried virgins).

Drunkenness or alcohol-associated delirium

A second group of conditions, two cases of delirium associated with alcoholic intoxication (among other examples in the corpus)[4] will illustrate the hyper- and hypoactive nuances that delirium can acquire. It is again the author of *Epidemics III* who comments on a Meliboean youth that ἐκ πότων καὶ ἀφροδισίων πολλῶν πολύν χρόνον θερμανθεὶς κατεκλίθη ('took to his bed with fever after

---

[4] López Salvá (1999: 523) offers a comprehensive study on drunkenness in the Hippocratic corpus, and Thumiger (2017: 226) lists several cases of alcohol consumption associated with mental problems.

indulging in drinking and sexual pleasures for a long time').[5] On the tenth day παρέκρουσεν ἀτρεμέως, ἦν δὲ κόσμιός τε καὶ σιγῶν ('he was delirious (*parekrouse*) but calm (*atremeôs*), rather well-behaved and quiet').[6] Later on, though, on the fourteenth day, his silence became irrational talk: παρέκρουσεν, πολλὰ παρέλεγεν ('delirious (*parekrousen*), much wandering talk (*parelegen*)').[7] Finally, on the twentieth day ἐξεμάνη, πολὺς βλησTρισμός ('agitation (*exemanê*), very restless').[8]

It is clear from the account that the author is describing a succession of repeated and limited episodes of impaired consciousness, where the boy was not his usual self. Even more explicit about the nature of impaired consciousness is a different case described by the author of *Epidemics IV*.

Ὁ πρῶτος παρενεχθείς, μειράκιον ... οὗτος παρέκρουσεν, οἶμαι ὀγδόῃ, τρόπον τὸν ἀκόλαστον, ἀνίστασθαι, μάχεσθαι, αἰσχρομυθεῖν ἰσχυρῶς, οὐ τοιοῦτος ἐών ... ὕπνος ἐγένετο ξυνεχής ... ἔπειτα ἐξεμάνη τε αὖτις καὶ ἀπέθανε ταχέως ἑνδεκαταῖος, προφάσιος οἶμαι πιεῖν ἄκρητον συχνὸν πρῖν ἐκμανῆναι ὀλίγῳ. *Epid. IV.15. LCL*: 102, 17; 20–1. 104, 1–3; 4–6.

The first affected by delirium (*parenechtheis*) was a lad ... He had, I think, on the eighth day the uncontrolled (*akolaston*) type of delirium (*parekrousen*): leaping up, fighting, and swearing a lot – although he was not that kind of person ... He developed continuous sleep ... Afterwards he was delirious (*exemanê*) again and suddenly died on the eleventh day. The cause (I believe): drinking abundant undiluted [wine] shortly before the frenzy (*ekmanênai*).

Of note in this passage are both the contrast that the writer highlights between the subject's usual character and his behaviour during the affection, as well as the constant changes in his levels of consciousness described. Indeed, his symptoms oscillate between impaired consciousness at the hyperactive side of the spectrum and sleep at the hypoactive one.

---

5 *Epid. III. CUF XVII.16*: Case 16–C16: 111, 10–12.
6 *Epid. III. CUF XVII.16*: Case 16–112: 7–8.
7 *Epid. III. CUF XVII.16*: Case 16–C16: 112, 10–11. There is a textual problem with παρέκρουσεν. Only one manuscript omitted it altogether, and this is Jouanna's choice. Most manuscripts present παρεκρούσθη, which the Teubner edition corrected to παρέκρουσεν. I agree with Jones (1923: 286), who also presents this reading. In this case παρέκρουσεν and παρέλεγεν do preserve their original and different (though complementary) meanings.
8 *Epid. III. CUF XVII.16*: Case 16–C16: 112, 12.

In terms of vocabulary, the author of *Epidemics III* uses *parakrouô* not only for describing calm impaired consciousness, but also the restless type. Furthermore, in this description, *ekmainomai* seems to denote – like *maniê* in the disease of the young virgins – a more intense nuance. Also, for the author of *Epidemics IV* the terms convey a similar ambiguity. In this account, *parakrouô* seems to be rephrasing *parapheromai* (another word associated with delirium), and the adverb *autis* (like *palin* earlier) suggests that *ekmainomai* is picking up the meaning of the former two. Namely, all three verbs are referring to a hyperactive type of delirium. In another chapter within the same book, however, the author explains that his patient was παραφερόμενος ἐξ ὕπνου, οὐκ ἐξεμάνη ('delirious (*parapheromenos*) after sleep, not agitated (*exemanê*)').[9] When collating all these elements, it appears that these authors acknowledged at least two types of delirium characterised by their behaviour as hypoactive (*atremeôs*) and hyperactive (*akolaston*), respectively, which they described with the same terminology.

Although strictly from a medical point of view, both cases seem like alcohol-associated affections rather than drunkenness, the acuteness (none of the processes prolong in time), the episodic nature as well as the constant fluctuations and changes in both excerpts suggest,[10] once again, remarkable swings within the intermediate areas of the spectrum of consciousness (which we would nowadays define as alterations in the level of consciousness and not mental illness). Moreover, the association with alcohol further reinforces this view, as there seems to be an element of intoxication to them.

Phrenitis

The last condition under scrutiny is broadly alluded to within the Hippocratic corpus and illustrates many of the above-discussed

---

[9] *Epid. IV.45. LCL:* 138, 18.
[10] Thumiger (2017: 222–4) acknowledges several of these features; however, because she uses a wide definition of mental illness that does not distinguish insanity from impaired consciousness, some of these nuances are lost (particularly when the Hippocratic texts are compared to Aretaeus).

phenomena. It should be emphasised that *phrenitis* was associated by the Hippocratic medical writers with a large array of symptoms[11] – particularly pain – among which delirium was only another element (and not always the most remarkable). Some nosological treatises that address it are particularly useful for catching a glimpse of what impaired consciousness must have looked like for these doctors. *Diseases I, II* and *III* (written by different authors) all address *phrenitis* and provide various and useful perspectives. Let us begin with *Diseases I*:

... παρανοέει τε ὤνθρωπος καὶ οὐκ ἐν ἑωυτῷ ἐστιν ... προσεοίκασι δὲ μάλιστα οἱ ὑπὸ τῆς φρενίτιδος ἐχόμενοι τοῖσι μελαγχολώδεσι κατὰ τὴν παράνοιαν· οἵ τε γὰρ μελαγχολώδεις ... καὶ παράνοοι γίνονται, ἔνιοι δὲ καὶ μαίνονται· καὶ ἐν τῇ φρενίτιδι ὡσαύτως· οὕτω δὲ ἧσσον ἡ μανίη τε καὶ ἡ παραφρόνησις γίνεται, ὅσῳπερ ἡ χολὴ τῆς χολῆς ἀσθενεστέρη ἐστίν. *Morb I. 30. LCL*: 158, 5–6; 9–11; 13–16.

... The person becomes delirious (*paranoeei*) and is no longer himself ... Patients with *phrenitis* most resemble those affected by black bile as regards their delirium (*paranoian*) ... Indeed, the latter also become delirious (*paranooi*), and some of them even have an outbreak of frenzy (*mainontai*). The same occurs to those affected by *phrenitis*, but both the frenzy (*maniê*) and the delirium (*paraphronêsis*) are less insofar as their bile is weaker than the [black] bile.

Interestingly, the writer interprets the state of the patient as 'not being himself', similar to the previous case, where the drunken boy 'was not that kind of person' (*Epid. IV.15. LCL*: 104, 1). This estrangement from the pre-existing characteristics of the sufferer helps the doctor in the diagnosis, which points towards an acute rather than chronic condition (when symptoms prolong in time it becomes more difficult to separate the baseline personality of the individual from the actual illness). Also important to remark is that *melancholia* is not yet a disease in its own right. The author is simply referring to individuals affected by black bile, as opposed to the bile that characterises *phrenitis*, which is weaker, and hence, so too the symptoms. Regarding the delirium terminology, the partial synonymy persists. The author uses *paranoeô-paranoia-paranoos* as equivalent to *paraphronêsis*, whereas *mainomai-maniê* – like

[11] McDonald (2009a).

ekmainomai in the Meliboean boy's description – seems to express a more extreme and hyperactive level of derangement.[12]

Other nosological treatises are more explicit about what the actual symptoms looked like, namely, they go into details about the nature of the impairment in *phrenitis*. *Diseases II* specifies that the patient φοβεῖται, καὶ δείματα ὁρᾷ καὶ ὀνείρατα φοβερὰ καὶ τοὺς τεθνηκότας ἐνίοτε ('is in panic and sees terrible things, frightening dreams and sometimes, even the dead').[13] Indeed, this is not completely different from the symptoms described for the young girls or the drunken lads. Ultimately, the writer is describing disturbing hallucinations.

The author of *Diseases III*, finally, presents us with a different kind of alteration in the hypoactive side of the spectrum of consciousness that he also associates with *phrenitis*:

... ἔκφρονές εἰσι, καὶ ἀτενὲς βλέπουσι, καὶ τἆλλα παραπλήσια ποιέουσι τοῖσιν ἐν τῇσι περιπλευμονίῃσιν, ὅταν ἔκφρονες ἔωσι. *Morb III.9. LCL*: 18, 22–4; 20, 1.

... they are delirious (*ekphrones*) and stare fixedly, and do the rest of the things in a similar way as those affected by *peripneumonia* when they become delirious (*ekphrones*).

These *phrenitic* patients seem to be suffering hypoactive impaired consciousness, for they do not move. Nowadays we would probably define this symptom as 'vigil coma', that is, a condition where individuals are completely disconnected from the environment, but with their eyes wide open.

It is remarkable that three different medical writers described rather different manifestations of *phrenitis*, which nonetheless defined, in their understanding, the same condition: various states of extreme hyper- and hypoactivity, along with diverse hallucinations, were all subsumed within the notion of *phrenitis*; in other words, one single condition that causes several variations of what we nowadays consider as impaired consciousness.

---

[12] Thumiger (2013: 72) has considered that all these *manié*- compounds have a 'superlative quality and represent a higher degree of insanity'. However, this nuance is not generalisable to the whole corpus. In *On the sacred disease* the author describes two forms of the ailment (a hyper- and a hypoactive one), and he claims that 'those who are delirious (*mainomenoi*) due to phlegm are quieter, neither do they shout nor are they agitated'. In other words, the term can also be used to describe a hypoactive behaviour.

[13] *Morb. II.72. LCL*: 326, 11–12.

A similar conclusion could be drawn from all three conditions that we have analysed. There is a set of related signs and symptoms, which are present in and characteristic of – but not exclusive to – certain unrelated conditions. This acute and short-lived clinical presentation has several similarities with our idea of delirium, but not necessarily of mental illness. As a matter of fact, the distinction between impaired consciousness and madness in the Hippocratic texts was not a major concern for the authors because they mostly disregarded madness and mainly focused on delirium.[14]

Symptoms, location, cause and treatment of delirium: the loose notion of disease in the Hippocratic Corpus

As highlighted above, impaired (or abnormal) perceptions and speech disorders – amid several other symptoms – are very characteristic of our current idea of wakeful impaired consciousness. When chasing these two major clinical manifestations across the subsequent authors and periods, it will become clear that not only ideas about impaired consciousness but also the understanding of the notion of disease among ancient doctors changed over time.

Undoubtedly, in the previous examples hallucinations were important for the Hippocratic doctors. The young girls ὁρῆν δοκέειν δαίμονάς τινας ἐφ᾽ ἑωυτῶν δυσμενέας ('think that they can see spirits hostile to them');[15] a *phrenitic* patient δείματα ὁρᾷ καὶ ὀνείρατα φοβερὰ καὶ τοὺς τεθνηκότας ἐνίοτε ('sees terrible things, frightening dreams and sometimes, even the dead');[16] and the author of *On the sacred disease* explains that when the brain is ill, μήτε τὴν ὄψιν ἀτρεμίζειν μήτε τὴν ἀκοήν, ἀλλ᾽ ἄλλοτε ἄλλα ὁρᾶν καὶ ἀκούειν ('neither sight, nor hearing remain still; instead sometimes we see or hear certain things, whereas at other times others').[17] It cannot be emphasised enough that these abnormal perceptions are framed in the texts as only one clinical finding among various others, such as fever, pain, abnormal movements

---

[14] Garofalo (1997, Introd: vii) goes as far as to posit that the Hippocratic doctors did not discuss chronic diseases at all.
[15] *Virg. CUF. I.1*: 188, 7–8.   [16] *Morb. II.72. LCL*: 326, 11–12.
[17] *Morb. Sacr. CUF 14.5*: 26, 15.

in the hands, photophobia, etc. We shall later see that their status and relevance in post-Hellenistic and Galenic accounts will increase.

On the other hand, speech disorders will suffer the exact opposite process: namely, they were consistently related to delirium in the Hippocratic collection, but their importance waned in later periods. Above is the example of Euryanax's young daughter, whose hypoactive delirium – described as *parelêrei*[18] – caused her to not talk. I have elsewhere mentioned several other cases where the symptom was so strongly related to this condition that the terminology denoting senseless talking was used interchangeably with delirium (as opposed to normal speech, which was utilised to convey the idea of lucidity).[19]

In terms of the bodily parts, although the *locus affectus* is a post-classical notion,[20] Padel has remarked that among the tragic poets, and also in the Hippocratic corpus, there are several attempts at associating states of altered consciousness with some *splachna* or 'innards'. In her insightful analysis, these were often identified with specific organs (heart, brain, liver, lungs), certain liquids (blood, bile) or airy substances (including the breath); they could also be assimilated to specific tissues (blood vessels, the diaphragm) or even to more abstract concepts (*thumos, menos, nous, psuchê*).[21] Regardless of their anatomic placement, which was different in different texts, they tended to be involved in or enabled feeling and thinking.

Accordingly, the author of *On the sacred disease* (*Morb. Sacr. 14.5*: 26, 14–15) attributes hallucinations to the brain, whereas in *On diseases of girls* the heart and the diaphragm as well as the poor state of the blood are responsible for similar phenomena.

---

[18] *Epid. III. CUF I.6*: Case 6–B6: 72, 2; 4; 7; 11–13. This statement contradicts many scholars' perceptions about *parelêreô* (Di Benedetto, 1986: 47; Thumiger, 2013: 75). They tend to relate it to the non-technical meaning of *lêreô*, and therefore they associate it with a chatty delirium or an inarticulate kind of speech. In this passage, however, it clearly has the opposite connotation. There is another similar example in *Epidemics I (Epid. I. CUF XXVII.13*: Case 13–A 13: 59, 10–12), where γλῶσσα ἠφώνει, δεξιὴ χείρ παρελύθη ... παρελήρει πάντα ('the tongue was speechless, her right hand paralysed ... she was completely delirious (*parelêrei*)'). Again, if she were speechless she could have hardly been delirious in a chatty way.
[19] Pelavski (2020: 21–2). [20] McDonald (2011: 63, 76). [21] Padel (1994: 39).

Symptoms, location, cause and treatment

... ὑπὸ δὲ τῆς περὶ τὴν καρδίην πιέξιος ἀγχόνας κραίνουσιν, ὑπὸ δὲ τῆς κακίης τοῦ αἵματος ἀλύων καὶ ἀδημονέων ὁ θυμὸς κακὸν ἐφέλκεται. ἕτερον δὲ καὶ φοβερὰ ὀνομάζει· καὶ κελεύουσιν ἄλλεσθαι καὶ καταπίπτειν ἐς φρέατα ἢ ἄγχεσθαι. *Virg. CUF II.3*: 190, 4–8.

... due to the compression around the heart, [girls] strangle themselves, due to the bad condition of their blood, the *thumos*, restless and in anguish, tempts them to another evil. Moreover, it [the *thumos*] mentions frightful [apparitions], which order them to leap and throw themselves down wells or to strangle themselves.[22]

What is interesting about this passage is the fact that the author relates specific symptoms to specific innards. Although he does not explain how the heart, the *thumos* or the state of the blood cause those hallucinations, there is a link between anatomical location and clinical manifestation, which approaches a description of our way of thinking about diseases. Similarly, according to *On breaths*, drunkenness is associated with changes in the blood:

πάλιν ἐν τῇσι μέθῃσι πλέονος ἐξαίφνης γενομένου τοῦ αἵματος μεταπίπτουσιν αἱ ψυχαὶ καὶ τὰ ἐν τῇσι ψυχῇσι φρονήματα, καὶ γίνονται τῶν μὲν παρεόντον κακῶν ἐπιλήσμονες, τῶν δὲ μελλόντων ἀγαθῶν εὐέλπιδες ... *Flat. CUF 14.3*: 122, 6–10.

Again, during heavy drinking, as blood suddenly becomes more abundant, the *psuchai* undergo change along with the *phronêmata* that are in them (in the *psuchai*). Hence, we become oblivious to our present miseries, and cheerful about a happy future ...

This excerpt is only mentioning mood changes. Nevertheless, if alcohol mainly affects the volume of blood, thereby compromising the *psuchai* – which seems to be the core implication of this passage – we can presume that the alterations of consciousness described in the examples of the young drinkers should also be attributed to similar occurrences.

Concerning *phrenitis*, finally, some Hippocratic texts consider it to be caused by bile. The discrepancy, though, emerges regarding

[22] The grammar of the last sentence is unclear: I considered θυμὸς to be the subject of the two verbs ἐφέλκεται ... δὲ καὶ ὀνομάζει. I disagree with Boubon's correction – ἑτεροῖα – and prefer the reading from the manuscripts (that is, ἕτερον), as though the author was suggesting that the evil enticed by the *thumos* was different from the one caused by the compressed heart. I translated κελεύουσιν in agreement with φοβερὰ because in the first passage of this treatise (mentioned in the chapter on delirium), the author hints that the frightful spirits (*daimones*) from the visions made patients strangle themselves.

where it causes the damage. The author of the nosological treatise *On affections* considers that ἡ δὲ νοῦσος γίνεται ὑπὸ χολῆς, ὅταν κινηθεῖσα πρὸς τὰ σπλάγχνα καὶ τὰς φρένας προσίζῃ ('the disease occurs due to bile, when it sets in motion and settles in the organs and the diaphragm (*ta splachna kai tas phrenas*)'),[23] whereas for the author of *On diseases I* it needs to enter the blood:

φρενῖτις δ' οὕτως ἔχει· τὸ αἷμα ἐν τῷ ἀνθρώπῳ πλεῖστον συμβάλλεται μέρος συνέσιος· ... ὅταν οὖν χολὴ κινηθεῖσα ἐς τὰς φλέβας καὶ ἐς τὸ αἷμα ἐσέλθῃ ... παρανοέει τε ὤνθρωπος καὶ οὐκ ἐν ἑωυτῷ ἐστιν. *Morb. I.30. LCL*: 158, 1–3; 6.

Phrenitis is like this: the blood in man accumulates most of his *sunesis* ... When bile sets in motion and enters the vessels and the blood ... the man suffers delirium and is no longer himself.

Ultimately, the debate that all these Hippocratic authors are having concerns their idea of mind and its localisation (which – as Padel points out – is not alien to the philosophical questions that the tragic poets were debating at the same time).[24]

As far as mechanisms and treatments are concerned, we have already caught small glimpses in the previous discussion: delirium in young virgins stemmed from an abnormal accumulation of blood that affected the heart and diaphragm due to obstructed drainage from the uterus. Not surprisingly, the author acknowledged that the release came when the discharge of blood stopped being obstructed.[25] The recommended treatment to achieve this, however, seems to be more related to sociological needs – he advised marriage and pregnancy – than to the biological mechanism that caused the disease.

In cases of drunkenness the author of *On breaths* mentioned the increase in the volume of blood, but neither blood-letting nor any other treatments are suggested.[26] Regarding *phrenitis*, as McDonald has pointed out, the therapeutic approach is fairly non-specific.[27] Authors tend to group the condition with other

---

[23] *Aff. 10. LCL*: 18, 19–20. Padel (1994: 13) considers the *phrenes* to be at the centre of the tragic language of mind, and the *splachna* as the general collection of innards.

[24] Padel (1994: 38–40).

[25] ὁκόταν μὴ ἐμποδίζῃ τι τοῦ αἵματος τὴν ἀπόρρυσιν. *Virg. CUF II.4*: 190, 15–16.

[26] This idea seems to be in line with the Heraclitean notion of a 'moist soul' associated with drunkenness, which Padel has explored (1994: 41).

[27] McDonald (2009a: 51–8).

diseases,[28] particularly with *peripneumonia* and *pleuritis*,[29] and recommend general treatments for specific symptoms. Purgation, (upwards and downwards),[30] warming (especially in the painful site) and drinks except for wine are recommended.[31] Interestingly pain is the doctors' main concern and the main target of their treatment. Unlike what we will see in the post-Hellenistic sources, there are almost no remedies specifically aimed at delirium. Only the author of *On affections* posits that λούειν δὲ πολλῷ καὶ θερμῷ κατὰ κεφαλῆς ἐν ταύτῃ τῇ νούσῳ συμφέρει· ... αὐτὸς αὑτοῦ ἐγκρατέστερος γίνεται ('it is convenient to bathe those suffering of this disease in abundant hot water from the head downwards ... for individuals become more in control of themselves').[32]

As we have seen, the articulation between symptoms, affected parts, pathophysiological mechanism and treatment is rather loose at best, or non-existent in most cases. There are very few accounts that link symptoms to affected parts, and there seems to be a complete divorce between therapeutic methods and physio-pathological mechanisms.[33] Consequently, it is safe to suggest that these doctors' notion of illness – compared to ours and to their successors – is rather loose. In other words, impaired consciousness in general and *phrenitis* in particular are framed as clusters of related symptoms not clearly bound to their triggering mechanism and need to be treated like other acute conditions, not too far from our own ideas about impaired consciousness, but quite different from our notion of disease.

---

[28] With other acute diseases (*Acut. CUF*: 5), with diseases of the cavity (*Aff. LCL*: 6).

[29] *Morb. III. LCL*: 15 and *Aff. LCL*: 10.

[30] *Morb. II. LCL*: 72, *Aff. LCL*: 10 and *Acut. CUF*: 23. Downward purgation is not explicitly a treatment for *phrenitis*, but for any acute disease with pain below the diaphragm.

[31] μηδ' οἶνον πινέτω ('he should not drink wine'), *Morb. II. LCL* 72: 110, 13–14; τοῦτον χλιαίνειν χλιάσμασιν ὑγροῖσι καὶ πώμασι πλὴν οἴνου ('this patient should be warmed with moist fomentations and with drinks other than wine'), *Morb. III. LCL* 9: 18, 5–6; and χλιαίνειν ἢν ὀδύνη ἔχῃ ... ποτῷ δὲ χρῆσθαι πλὴν οἴνου τῶν ἄλλων ὅτῳ ἂν θέλῃς ('warm him if he is in pain ... in terms of drinks, it is necessary to give him anything you want except for wine'), *Aff. LCL 10*: 18, 12–14.

[32] *Aff. LCL 10*: 18, 17–18; 20.

[33] I disagree in this sense with McDonald (2009a: 52–3), who considers that downwards purgation is aimed at removing the excess of bile. There is no explicit mention of it. Actually, purgation of the lower cavity is one among other general measures to treat *peripneumonia* and any acute disease (whether it is caused by bile or not).

CHAPTER 4

DELIRIUM, MADNESS AND DISEASE AMONG POST-HELLENISTIC AUTHORS

Among the post-Hellenistic sources the opposition impaired consciousness–mental illness becomes more explicit. Modern scholars, however, have persevered in ignoring impaired consciousness. As far as the notion of disease is concerned, the different components that we have seen as barely theoretically related in the Hippocratic corpus will be more strongly linked among these authors.

Celsus

Celsus' *On medicine* offers a good example of the above. It has triggered abundant discussion about madness where scholars have completely ignored consciousness.[1] The reason for this omission is that the modern debate tends to focus on *insania* as a whole but disregards the context in which it appears, especially the relations that the author establishes with the conditions addressed in the subsequent chapters. Indeed, Celsus presents delirium within a system of oppositions that aims at distinguishing it from mental illness, on the one hand, and from other forms of impaired consciousness, on the other.

The whole discussion is presented in the first part of the nosology section of *On medicine* (book 3). In it, chapter 18 tackles *insania*, an umbrella-term comprised of three nosological entities. Although a superficial reading might suggest that they are equally relevant, the first of them – *phrenesis* – has a different status. Not only does it take up most of the explanation, but it is also the only

---

[1] Specifically focused on madness in *On medicine* is Pigeaud's paper (1994: 257–79). Stok proposes a more comprehensive history of mental disease in antiquity and devotes an important section of it to Celsus (1996: 2331–41). Again, both authors – and also Gourevitch (1991: 561–6) – address vocabulary issues and explore correspondences with the Hippocratic corpus; however, none of them considers consciousness.

one explicitly referred to by its name, and whose relations to other conditions are clearly established.

Phrenesis is initially contrasted with the second and third types of *insania* – possibly *melancholia* and *mania*, which we would nowadays classify as mental illness[2] – and subsequently, it is the only one of the three emphatically opposed to the conditions addressed in the following chapters, namely, *cardiacum*[3] and *lethargy*.[4] *siquidem mens in illis labat, in hoc constat* ('While in [*phrenesis*] the *mens*[5] gives in, in [*cardiacum*] it endures'),[6] and *in eo difficilior somnus, prompta ad omnem audaciam mens est: in hoc marcor et inexpugnabilis paene dormiendi necessitas* ('whereas in [*phrenesis*] sleeping is more difficult, and the *mens* is prone to any kind of insolence; in [*lethargy*] there is torpor and an almost overpowering need of sleep').[7] It should be highlighted that the latter two diseases are the closest ancient equivalents to the other prototypes of impaired consciousness that I have chosen. As a matter of fact, among the post-Hellenistic writers *phrenitis* became the prototypical example of wakeful impaired consciousness, *lethargy* of drowsy impaired consciousness and *cardiacum* of total loss of consciousness.

---

[2] Stok (1996: 2317), and also Pigeaud (1994: 257), take it for granted that the second and the third kinds of *insania* correspond to *melancholia* and *mania*, respectively. It is a likely hypothesis, but Celsus never states it explicitly. On the other hand, there are some contradictory hints regarding *melancholia*: it certainly is elsewhere associated with *bilis atra quam* μελαγχολίαν *appellant* ('black bile, which [the Greeks] call *melancholia*', *Med. 2.1*: 6), and black bile does cause *longa tristitia, cum longo timore et vigilia* ('prolonged sadness, fear and wakefulness', *Med. 2.7*: 22); however, on the list of spring diseases, *melancholia* is mentioned along with *insania*, as two different and independent nosological entities.

[3] *His morbis praecipue contrarium est id genus, quod cardiacum a Graecis nominatur, quamvis saepe ad eum phrenetici transeunt* ('The disease that the Greeks call *cardiacum* is particularly opposed to this one [*insania*], although *phrenetic* patients often evolve into it', *Med. 3.19*: 1).

[4] *Alter quoque morbus est aliter phrenetico contrarius* ('There is also an additional disease that differs from *phrenesis* in another way', *Med. 3.20*: 1).

[5] I will avoid translating the terms that refer to HOFs both in Latin and in Greek, because their rendering depends on interpretation. A good example is found with the Greek Hippocratic terminology: *gnômê* is translated by Mann (*Art.* 2012: 62) as 'mind', by Gundert (2000: 26) as 'judgement', by Jones (1931: 250) as 'intelligence' and by Craik (*Glan.* 2009: 77) as 'intellect'. My argument is that they were different forms of designating HOFs, therefore I will transliterate them, and only provide an English rendering when there is a clear nuance implied.

[6] *Med. 3.19*: 1. [7] *Med. 3.20*: 1.

The fact that Celsus feels the need to contrast only the first type of *insania* – that is, *phrenesis* – to these other forms of impaired consciousness constitutes a hint that such conditions were some-how related, or at least easily confused (whereas the second and third types of *insania* were perceived as more distinct entities).

The strongest hint to relate *phrenesis* to delirium, however, comes from the distinction among the different kinds of *insania*. Differential diagnosis between these three entities is based on the presence of fever, the length of the condition and some specific symptoms, particularly hallucinations. Indeed, the first kind of *insania*, *phrenesis*, *et acuta et in febre est* ('both acute and with fever'), and causes deceptive apparitions (*vanas imagines*) to which the *mens* surrenders.[8] These patients can be *alii tristes sunt; alii hilares; alii facilius continentur ... alii consurgunt et violenter quaedam manu faciunt ...* ('sad, others cheerful, some are easily controlled ... and some resist and act violently').[9] The second *genus* of *insania* oppresses for a 'longer period because it usually begins without fever' and 'consists of sadness that black bile seems to bring about'.[10] The third kind, finally, is the 'longest of all. So much so that it does not even compromise life, for it tends to occur in strong bodies'.[11] Some of the affected patients are 'deceived not by their *mens*, but by *imagines* like those perceived – according to the poets – by Ajax or Orestes, when they were insane', whereas in others 'the *animus* becomes void of understanding'.[12] In this description (that is, in the characterisa-tion of the second type of the third form of *insania*), *mens*, *animus* and *consilium* are used interchangeably.

The acute nature of *phrenesis*, the presence of fever and the various kinds of hallucinations (*vanas imagines*) that cause all sorts of disturbed behaviour – that is, impaired responsiveness – once the *mens* gives in to them, make it easy for us to identify it with the Hippocratic *phrenitis*, and therefore with a condition

[8] *Med. 3.18*: 1.   [9] *Med. 3.18*: 3.
[10] *spatium longius recipit, quia fere sine febre incipit ... consistit in tristitia, quam videtur bilis atra contrahere* (*Med. 3.18*: 17).
[11] *ex his longissimum, adeo ut vitam ipsam non impediat; quod robusti corporis esse consuevit* (*Med. 3.18*: 19).
[12] *imaginibus, non mente falluntur, quales insanientem Aiacem vel Orestem percepisse poetae ferunt: quidam animo desipiunt* (*Med. 3.18*: 19).

where (wakeful) loss of consciousness predominates. These coincidences notwithstanding, it should be noted that Celsus, probably influenced by the ongoing debates, feels the need to distinguish between this condition and others that no Hippocratic writer mentions (at least not as such, even accepting the leading hypothesis in scholarship that the second and third kinds of *insania* correspond to *mania* and *melancholia*, respectively).[13] Beyond the lack of fever and the more chronic course of the second and third subtypes, Celsus finds the cognitive disturbances themselves to be distinct in each condition. Whilst *phrenesis* can trigger virtually any kind of hallucination (thereby affecting connectedness to the environment) and compromise responsiveness (as any episode of delirium does), the other two are more stereotypical. The variant caused by black bile can only produce pathological sadness, whereas patients with the third type of *insania* either have their *animus* compromised or suffer from *imagines*. Yet, the latter are different from those caused by *phrenesis* because they do not affect the *mens*. Judging by what we know about Ajax and Orestes, we can suppose that those apparitions resemble what we would nowadays define as a structured delusion, that is, a condition where reasoning is preserved but the patient holds elaborated beliefs and ideas, which are stable in time and not shared by the others (quite different from the more chaotic thought disorders of acute deliriums).

According to Stok, *On medicine* is the first extant medical text where these three 'psychiatric' conditions appear related.[14] Beyond the fact that *phrenesis* is *stricto sensu* not a psychiatric condition, it is likely that the discussion of these three illnesses and their distinction was very much part of the post-Hellenistic debate. A hint to support this hypothesis can be found in the pseudo-Galenic *Introduction* (*Eisagogê*). Although the compiler of this introductory handbook discusses *phrenitis* among acute diseases, and *melancholia* and *mania* among the chronic ones, he

---

[13] For the Hippocratic medical writers *mania* was a symptom and not a disease in its own right (Pigeaud 1981: 100–1). Regarding *melancholia*, even though it is mentioned in several texts (in some even related to *phrenitis*, *Morb. I.30. LCL*: 178, 15–16), its nature remains fairly vague.
[14] Stok (1996: 2324).

defines *phrenitis* as ἔκστασις διανοίας μετὰ παρακοπῆς σφοδρᾶς ('disruption (*ekstasis*) of the *dianoia* with strong delirium (*parakopê*)'),[15] and the other two – which are different forms (*eidê*) of the same illness – as περὶ τὴν διάνοιαν ἐκστάσεως ('*dianoia* disrupted (*ekstaseôs*)').[16] Considering the coincidence in terminology, it is not unlikely that these diseases were perceived as related entities, and it was the dichotomous classification (acute versus chronic) which prevented the author from discussing them together.[17] In other words, the difficulty of separating acute delirium from chronic mental illness is evidenced in other post-Hellenistic works.

In summary, according to Celsus, wakeful impaired consciousness is described in opposition to other forms of impaired consciousness (*cardiacum* and *lethargy*); it is contrasted to mental illness (second and third types of *insania*), and presented as an array of acute symptoms that change substantially during their course. As I will argue, the notion of disease that emerges from Celsus' approach to delirium is strongly influenced by this system of oppositions.

Celsus and the notion of disease

From the large Hippocratic list of symptoms that characterised *phrenitis*, in *On medicine* the emphasis has patently shrunk to abnormal perceptions, which have become the key diagnostic finding. Most of the discussion, in fact, is aimed at describing how those *vanas imagines* and their effects on behaviour are useful in distinguishing *phrenesis* from the other forms of *insania*. This symptom in particular (and to a lesser extent the presence of fever and the length of the ailment) are used by Celsus to draw contrasts between the three types of conditions.

On the other hand, contrary to this increased pre-eminence of hallucinations in the discussions, the other symptom that was

---

[15] *Int. CUF 13.9*: 51, 4–5.   [16] *Int. CUF 13.24*: 57, 6–7.
[17] This idea is further reinforced by the *Medical definitions*, another didactic treatise, which describes *phrenitis* as παρακοπὴ διανοίας ... καὶ διανοίας ἔκστασις (*Def. Med.* 234. *K.XIX*: 412, 17–18), and *mania* as ἔκστασις τῆς διανοίας (*Def. Med.* 246. *K.XIX*: 416, 8). In this text, however, *melancholia* is defined with different terminology.

Celsus

ubiquitous in Hippocratic descriptions of delirium, speech disorders, has become less relevant (even if they are still present
and often associated with delirium). In book 2 (which addresses
generalities about diseases) Celsus describes how in *insania* with
fever one should expect patients to be *expeditior alicuius, quam
sani fuit, sermo subitaque loquacitas orta est, et haec ipsa sermo
audacior* ('more chatty than when healthy, and such sudden talk-
ativeness is often more aggressive').[18] Afterwards, when he characterises *phrenesis* he defines this symptom as *loqui aliena* (*Med.
3.18*: 2) – a calque of the Hippocratic *allophassein* (*Mul. I.41.
LCL*: 104, 3) – which he later on paraphrases as *intra verba
desipere* (*Med. 3.18*: 3), and *stulte dicere* (*Med. 3.18*: 11). It
seems that Celsus does still conceive a close association between
delirium and incoherent speech,[19] but it is much less frequently
mentioned than among the Hippocratic doctors.

Also relevant to this system of opposing symptoms is the emergence of wakefulness or sleep disturbances as a characteristic sign
of *phrenesis*, paralleled by the association between *lethargy* and
drowsiness (mentioned above). This appears to be a post-Hellenistic
addition,[20] for such difficulty in falling asleep is not mentioned in
any of the Hippocratic treatises that describe *phrenitis*.

In terms of bodily location, several of the obscure and vaguely
defined Hippocratic innards are re-elaborated in later texts as
distinct *loci affecti*. The *Anonymus Parisinus* posits that for
Erasistratus *phrenitis* originated in the meninx, for Praxagoras
in the heart and for Diocles in the diaphragm.[21] It could be
argued that this wide variety of locations started to shrink, and
towards the post-Hellenistic era the debate was predominantly
dichotomous, namely encephalocentric against cardiocentric

[18] *Med. 2.7*: 24. Stok (1996: 2334) has related this passage to a Hippocratic ἐκ κοσμίου θρασεῖα ἀπόκρισις κακόν (*Prorrh. I. 44. LCL*).
[19] A particularly explicit example appears in the discussion of gangrene (within the pharmacological section): *alii quamvis mentis suae compotes sunt, balbutiendo tamen vix sensus suos explicant* ('the others [patients with gangrene and fever], although they are in full control of their *mens*, nonetheless, stammering, they can hardly express their feelings,' *Med 5.26*: 14E). The emphatic concession *quamvis ... tamen* highlights that in Celsus' conception it was unusual to see cases with speech problems and no delirium.
[20] A similar link can be found in the *Anonymus Parisinus* (*Anon. Paris. I.2, 3–4*: 4, 2–3; 8–9) and, as we shall later discuss, also in Aretaeus and in Galen.
[21] *Anon. Paris. I.1, 1–3*: 2, 3–12.

41

views. Celsus' choice in this respect gives testimony of his harmonising stance towards conflicting views. It was not at all an innocent choice that he tackled *phrenesis* among other diseases that affect the entire body. In this way he did not have to commit to any of the positions, but at the same time did not have to challenge them either. I do not completely agree with Pigeaud's remark that Celsus based his classification of diseases on the *locus affectus*, thereby disregarding the opposition acute–chronic.[22] In the case of *insania*, this indefinite location in the body is shared by all three forms of the disease, thereby uniting rather than separating them. On the contrary, their length is actually one of the factors that distinguishes them from one another (perhaps his 'somehow in the middle' attitude prevented Celsus from strictly defining them as acute or chronic, yet the time frame is crucial in his descriptions).[23] To a certain extent, we could posit that this 'middle way' was his form of navigating the strict oppositions imposed by the post-Hellenistic binary classification scheme. He managed to avoid positioning himself among either the encephalocentrics or the cardiocentrics, and at the same time he got away from the sharp distinction of acute versus chronic, although he did acknowledge the importance of the length of the conditions.

Pathophysiological mechanisms are often omitted in *On medicine*, and the treatment tends to be symptomatic and mostly based on post-Hellenistic sources. In this regard, Celsus mentions the ancients only once (*Med. 3.18*: 5), while he persistently juxtaposes different opinions with Asclepiadean practices (*Med. 3.18*: 5, 6, 14, 15). Even if some therapies suggested can be linked to allusions in the Hippocratic corpus, their use has evidently triggered larger debates during this period. A good example is the discussion about the convenience of light versus

---

[22] Pigeaud (1994: 275). It is undeniable that such a distinction relates *On medicine* to the medico-doxographical tradition of the *loci affecti* (van der Eijk, 1999: 322), albeit a none-too-committed one.

[23] Some affections were difficult to fit within this dichotomous division, as Celsus himself acknowledges (*Med. 3*: 2–3). Also, other authors had incorporated intermediate categories (in *Medical definitions* there are acute, hyperacute, chronic and intermediate, *Def. Med.* 138–42. *K.XIX*: 388–99, respectively).

darkness for these patients:[24] Celsus contrasts the opinion of the ancients – *tales aegros in tenebris habebant, eo quod iis contrarium esset exterreri* ('to keep such patients in darkness, for it is counterproductive to have them frightened') – with that of Asclepiades – *tanquam tenebris ipsis terrentibus, in lumine habendos eos dixit* ('because darkness is terrifying they should be kept in luminous places he said')[25] – and opts, in a clear example of his encyclopaedic method, for the middle way (that is, he recommends allowing the patient to choose light or darkness according to his preference). The *Anonymus Parisinus* parallels in a much more succinct manner both the opposing points of view and the uncommitted conclusion (*Anon. Paris. I.3, 1*: 4, 18–21), thereby confirming that the matter was being debated.

Other treatments are completely foreign to the Hippocratic collection, but rather common in post-Hellenistic sources. Such is the case with therapies using the spoken word,[26] flogging and restraints,[27] and sleep-inducing drugs. Given that one of the dichotomous oppositions to distinguish *phrenesis* from *lethargy* is its wakefulness, Celsus recommends poppy (*papaver*) (*Med. 3.18*: 12), which amongst a few other options, was popular in post-Hellenistic treatises to achieve sleep.[28]

---

[24] It is likely that such a controversy originated from a passage in *On diseases II*, where the phrenitic patient τὸ φῶς φεύγει καὶ τοὺς ἀνθρώπους, καὶ τὸ σκότος φιλέει, καὶ φόβος λάζεται ('avoids light and people, loves darkness and is seized by fear', *Morb. II. LCL* 72: 110, 2–4).

[25] *Med 3.18*: 5.

[26] *interdum etiam elicienda ipsius intentio; ut fit in hominibus studiosis litterarum …* ('Occasionally patients' interest should be awakened, like in men who are fond of literature… *Med. 3.18*:11.) Similar examples appear in *Anon. Paris. I.3, 6*: 6, 16–24 and, as we shall later see, in Aretaeus.

[27] *… eos, qui violentius se gerunt, vincire convenit, ne vel sibi vel alteri noceant … Quorundam audacia coercenda est … in quibus continendis plagae quoque adhibentur …* ('it is convenient to restrain those who behave violently, so that they neither hurt themselves nor the others … Their insolence should be controlled, … in them repressive blows can be applied. *Med 3.18*: 4, 10).

I have elsewhere argued (Pelavski: 2023) that the emphasis on these controversial treatments, which appear not only in *On medicine* but also in the *Anonymus Parisinus* (*Anon. Paris. I.3, 11*: 8, 26–8), and in Caelius Aurelianus' treatise (*Aur. Acut. I.65*), are likely related to the legal implications of impaired consciousness, especially to the liability of the carers.

[28] *Anon. Paris. I.3, 7*: 6, 25–6.

Of note is the fact that Celsus does not mention any patho-physiological mechanism for *phrenesis*.[29] As a result, the treatment is unrelated to the workings of the body and the disease, and it only targets symptoms, which it aims at counteracting. Naturally, because hallucinations and wakefulness have become the most prominent symptoms in this period, most remedies are aimed at controlling them. In other words, Celsus' strategy opposes each specific manifestation (represses aggressive cases, sedates the wakeful, offers light or darkness depending on their needs, etc.). Unlike the Hippocratic doctors, whose therapeutic approaches were aimed at several related diseases, Celsus describes a specific treatment that is exclusively meant for *phrenesis*. In this way, Celsus offers a particular and separate list of procedures for each of the different types of *insania*.

It could be argued, therefore, that the notion of illness in Celsus is less loose than amongst the Hippocratic doctors. He does not link the treatment to the causes and mechanisms but he does describe a specific combination of therapies that are linked to the specific symptoms and are unique to a particular disease (*phrenesis*).

Aretaeus

Like Celsus, Aretaeus' work supports the post-Hellenistic view of impaired consciousness and mental illness as easily confusable phenomena that needed to be separated through opposing features.[30] His attempts at distinguishing *phrenitis* from *melancholia* and *mania* are proof of this.[31] Regrettably, only the chapter

---

[29] Actually, the only statement in this respect refers to the relation between the second type of *insania* and black bilé: *consistit in tristitia, quam videtur bilis atra contrahere* ('it consists of sadness, which black bile seems to produce', *Med. 3.18*: 17).

[30] There is consensus in scholarship to consider *phrenitis*, *melancholia* and *mania* as paradigmatic examples of mental illness. This is the case of Pigeaud's chapter in his book devoted to madness in antiquity (1987: 71–94), of Murphy's dissertation (2013) and of McDonald's paper (2009a) and dissertation (2009b), which provide an in-depth description of *phrenitis*. In this way, much like with the Hippocratic corpus and Celsus' encyclopaedia, scholarship tends to overlook impaired consciousness, and *phrenitis* is seldom opposed to other entities.

[31] I disagree with Murphy (2013: 24–7), who sees in each disease a different kind of madness.

on the cure of *phrenitis* is extant (unlike the one on causes and symptoms); therefore, most conclusions will be based on passages drawn from it, as well as on various scattered allusions that Aretaeus made when he addressed other conditions.

οἵδε [οἱ φρενιτικοί] μὲν γὰρ παραισθάνονται, καὶ τὰ μὴ παρεόντα ὀρέουσι δῆθεν ὡς παρεόντα, καὶ τὰ μὴ φαινόμενα ἄλλῳ κατ᾽ ὄψιν ἰνδάλλεται. οἱ δὲ μαινόμενοι ὀρέουσι μόνως ὡς χρὴ ὁρῆν οὐ γιγνώσκουσι δὲ περὶ αὐτέων ὡς χρὴ γιγνώσκειν. *SD I.6. CMG (H).III*: 43, 1–4.

Phrenitics are subjected to misperceptions, and they see whatever is not present as though it was, and whatever is not apparent for somebody else, does appear in their sight. *Maniacs*, on the other hand, see what there is to see, but they do not recognise about it what needs to be recognised.

This passage offers a clear distinction between the cognitive impairment that characterises *phrenitis*, as opposed to the one that occurs among *maniacs* (and also *melancholics*, whom – like the author of the pseudo-Galenic *Introduction* – Aretaeus considered to be suffering from a different form of the same disease, *SD I.3. CMG (H).III*: 39, 28). In *phrenitis*, the abnormal behaviour is a consequence of impaired perceptions or disturbed connectedness (namely the hallucinations) but alertness is preserved, whereas in the others connectedness to the environment is intact, and the primary problem is their altered responsiveness due to impairment in their judgement. Generally speaking, both *melancholia* and *mania* present an altered responsiveness that manifests as abnormal behaviours, extreme emotions and delusions. Unlike the *phrenitic* delirium, these delusions are structured and persistent beliefs, which are not prompted by wrong perceptions, but by bad judgement (alertness is damaged).[32] Examples abound: those who mistrust remedies (*SD I.5. CMG (H).III*: 40, 1–2); the person who believed himself to be a brick and avoided water for fear of dissolving (*SD I.6. CMG (H).III*: 42, 19–20); the builder who could not be away from the building site (*SD I.6. CMG (H).III*: 42, 20–9); mystic delusions involving

---

[32] According to our modern conceptualisation, these conditions are presented as a mirror image of each other: *phrenitis* is presented as disturbed connectedness with preserved alertness, whereas *mania/melancolia* are defined as compromised alertness with undisturbed connectedness.

self-mutilation ordered by the gods (*SD I.6. CMG (H).III*: 43, 40–1; 44, 1), etc. It should be noted, however, that within these chronic conditions there are some specific moments where the author seems to be describing an acute delirium: μετεξέτεροι δὲ καὶ παραισθάνονται, παραφορῇ τῆς αἰσθήσιος ('some suffer from illusory perceptions and disturbances in their senses').[33] Nevertheless, this is still consistent with our understanding of mental illness, where some phases of acute psychosis can occur.

There is yet another clear delimitation between the domain of wakeful impaired consciousness/delirium and delusion when Aretaeus defines *mania*:

ἐκφλέγει γὰρ καὶ οἶνος ἐς παραφορὴν ἐν μέθῃ ἐκμαίνει δὲ καὶ τῶν ἐδεστῶν μετεξέτερα, ἢ μανδραγόρη, ἢ ὑοσκύαμος, ἀλλ' οὔ τί πω μανίη τάδε κικλήσκεται. ἐπὶ γὰρ σχεδίου γιγνόμενα καθίσταται θᾶττον τὸ δὲ ἔμπεδον ἡ μανίη ἴσχει. τῇδε τῇ μανίῃ οὐδέν τι ἴκελον ἡ λήρησις, γήραος ἡ ξυμφορή. *SD I.6. CMG (H).III*: 41, 15–19.

The wine excites [one] towards delirium (*paraphorên*) during drunkenness; certain foodstuffs also cause frenzy such as mandrake or henbane, yet this would never be called *mania* (for having appeared suddenly, they subside fast, whereas *mania* persists for a long time). Neither does *mania* resemble senility (*lêrêsis*), a mishap of old age.

In this passage, beyond the longer duration of *mania* – which is implicit in its classification as a chronic disease – Aretaeus uses the same delirium vocabulary that he had used in *phrenitis* to refer to intoxications with wine and psychoactive herbs (*paraphorê*, *ekmainei*).[34] Again, like the young lads from the Hippocratic corpus, drunkenness seems to be – at least terminologically – close to *phrenitis*. Moreover, not only should *mania* be distinguished from these acute forms of wakeful impaired consciousness, but it also differs from *lêrêsis*. This condition (which we would nowadays probably consider as akin to dementia) has become a nosological entity in its own right, where there is αἰσθήσιος γάρ ἐστι νάρκη καὶ

---

[33] *CD I.5. CMG (H).VII*: 157, 3–4.
[34] I disagree with Pigeaud's understanding of the wide 'field of madness', from which the doctors had to distribute the symptoms into three entities, namely *phrenitis*, *mania* and *melancholia* (1987: 80–1). It emerges from the text that *phrenitis* was envisaged by Aretaeus as a distinct condition, whereas the other two were different forms of the same illness.

Aretaeus

γνώμης νάρκωσις ἠδὲ. τοῦ νοῦ ὑπὸ ψύξιος ('numbing of perception and altered *gnômê* or *nous* due to coldness').[35]

Aretaeus and the concept of disease

Let us now explore the notion of disease that emerges from the account of delirium. If we take a closer look at the description, Aretaeus' understanding of the role of hallucinations goes one step further than Celsus': altered perceptions are not only at the centre of the diagnosis of *phrenitis*, but their compromise is the cause that triggers the whole process.

ὀξυήκοοι γὰρ ἠδὲ ψόφου καθαπτόμενοι φρενιτικοί ἀτὰρ ὑπὸ τῶνδε μαίνονται ... ἐρεθιστικὸν γὰρ τοιχογραφίη. καὶ γὰρ πρὸ τῶν ὀφθαλμῶν ἀμφαιρέουσί τινα ψευδέα ἰνδάλματα, καὶ τὰ μὴ ἐξίσχοντα ἀμφαφόωσι ὡς ὑπερίσχοντα ... ἀστεργὴς γὰρ τοῖσι νεύροισι ἡ σκληρὴ κοίτη. οὐχ ἥκιστα δὲ τῶν ἄλλων τοῖσι φρενιτικοῖσι τὰ νεῦρα πονέει ... μῦθοι καὶ λαλιὴ μὴ θυμοδακεῖς πάντα γὰρ εὐθυμέεσθαι χρή, μάλιστα τοῖσι ἐς ὀργὴν ἡ παραφορή ... ἢν γὰρ πρὸς τὴν αὐγὴν ἀγριαίνωσι, καὶ ὁρέωσι τὰ μὴ ὄντα, καὶ τὰ μὴ ὑπεόντα φαντάζωνται, ἢ ἀνθ᾽ ἑτέρων ἕτερα γιγνώσκωσι, ἢ ξένα ἰνδάλματα προβάλλωνται, καὶ τὸ ξύνολον τὴν αὐγὴν ἢ τὰ ἐν αὐγῇ δεδίττωνται, ζόφον αἱρέεσθαι χρή ἢν δὲ μὴ, τοὐναντίον. *CA I. CMG (H).V:* 91, 16–17; 18–20; 24–5; 92, 1–2, 3–7.

Because their hearing is sharp, *phrenitic* patients are sensitive to noise; in fact they become maddened by it ... They are irritated by [decorative] paintings on walls. Indeed, they perceive in front of their eyes some false images, and reach to touch things that are actually not sticking out as though they were protruding ... A hard bed is intolerable for their nerves: more than anything else, the nerves suffer amongst *phrenitic* patients ... The topics of the conversations [with the visitors] should not be upsetting. It is necessary to cheer them completely. Especially those whose delirium tends towards anger ... If they are annoyed by light because they see what does not exist, and imagine what has no underlying reality, or in front of different realities they interpret things differently, or alien images assault them, or they are frightened by the light or by what [they can see] in the light, then darkness should be chosen. Otherwise, the opposite.

It seems that *phrenitis* affects mainly the nerves and the senses (the *aisthêseis*), especially the sight through visual hallucinations, but also hearing and touch become particularly sensitive. So much so that sufferers *mainontai* due to noises, and a hard bed is *astergês* for them because the nerves are compromised. Even the abnormal

---

[35] *SD VI.6. CMG (H).III:* 41, 20–1.

47

movements of the hands (the *karphologia* and *krokudismos*),[36] which the Hippocratic authors had considered to be independent signs, in Aretaeus' description are framed as a consequence of the abnormal perceptions that make patients want to touch what does not really exist (these interpretations take for granted that reasoning was not affected in these cases). In this way, delirium (*mainontai, paraphorê*) is conceived primarily as a disturbance in sense perception (*oxuêkooi, pseudea/xena indalmata, phantazôntai* – that is, impaired connectedness to the environment), which leads to aggressive behaviour or hyperactive responsiveness (*erethistikon, es orgên, agriainôsi, dedittôntai*).[37]

On the other hand, there are no allusions to the other symptom that we have been chasing throughout the different sources. Speech disorders are virtually absent from this account of delirium. Only some changes, *phthenxin exallasôntai* (*CA I.1. CMG (H).V*: 94, 2), seem to be an occasional accompanying symptom but not an integral part of the syndrome. As commented above, even the term *lêrêsis* – often identified with speech disturbances in the Hippocratic collection – seems to have lost most of its previous connotations and has become an independent disease, which – furthermore – presents 'numbing of perceptions', thereby highlighting their relevance in this author's conception.[38]

To finish with Aretaeus' symptomatic components of delirium, he also presents the association of *phrenitis* with wakefulness (in perfect opposition to *lethargy* and drowsiness, as we have seen in Celsus and other post-Hellenistic authors: γὰρ πάννυχοι μὲν

---

[36] These symptoms are often described in ancient texts associated with delirium. They are characterised as abnormal automatic movements of the hands and fingers trying to pick up or grasp imaginary objects emerging from the walls, the clothes or the bed linen. As Walshe points out (2016: 100), it was usually associated with impaired consciousness.

[37] However, equating *paraphorê* with *paraisthanomai* would be a mistake. There are situations where misperceptions and hallucinations do not trigger bizarre behaviours (altered responsiveness). Such is the case of the aura that precedes *epileptic* attacks (a condition that we currently do consider as impaired consciousness), where neither the vocabulary, nor the description suggest delirium: κύκλῳ μαρμαρυγαὶ πρὸ τῆς ὄψιος πορφυρέων ἢ μελάνων, ἢ πάντων ὁμοῦ συμμεμιγμένων . . . ἠχοὶ ὤτων, βαρυοδμίη ('some round flashing sparks appear in front of their eyes; purple or black or all of the colours equally mixed . . . there is ringing in their ears, intense smells', *SA I.5. CMG (H).I*: 3, 9–12).

[38] *SD I.6. CMG (H).III*: 41, 20.

Aretaeus

ἐγρήσσωσι, μηδὲ δι' ἡμέρης εὕδωσι, ... βλησστρίζωνται δὲ καὶ ἐξανιστῶνται ('they are awake all night, and cannot sleep during the day ... and toss about and wake up').[39] Aretaeus' approach to the debates about the organs compromised in *phrenitis* is particularly illustrative of his lax eclectic method. The *loci affecti* include the nerves: τοῖσι φρενιτικοῖσι τὰ νεῦρα πονέει ('the nerves suffer in *phrenitic* patients');[40] the head and perceptions: τὸ δὲ κῦρος ἐν τοῖσι σπλάγχνοισί ἐστι ἐπὶ μανίῃ καὶ μελαγχολίῃ, ὅκωσπερ ἐν τῇ κεφαλῇ καὶ τοῖσι αἰσθήσεσι τὰ πολλὰ τοῖσι φρενιτικοῖσι ('the origin is in the organs (*splachnoisi*) in cases of *mania* and *melancholia*, as it is mostly in the head and the perceptions among *phrenitics*');[41] the *hypochondria*:[42] ἢν ἐξ ὑποχονδρίων καὶ μὴ ἀπὸ κεφαλῆς ἡ νοῦσος ᾖ. ἐνθάδε γὰρ τῆς ζωῆς ἐστι ἡ ἀρχή ('if the disease [*phrenitis*] comes from the *hypochondria* and not from the head (indeed, in them the origin of life resides');[43] and thoracic organs, including the heart and the lungs: ἐπεὶ δὲ καὶ θώρηκα ... ξὺν κραδίῃ καὶ πνεύμονι [in some patients, delirium originates from certain organs] 'in the thorax ... with the heart and lungs'.[44] Of note is the fact that Aretaeus always talks about the head (*kephalê*) and never about the brain (*enkephalos*) or its components (such as the meninges or the ventricles).[45] Nevertheless, we can still find in his descriptions – *mutatis mutandis* – a certain 'family resemblance' with Hellenistic theories about the nervous system, in that the nerves originate in the head and are related to perception: κεφαλὴ δὲ χῶρος μὲν αἰσθήσιος καὶ νεύρων ἀφέσιος ('the

---

[39] *CA I.1. CMG (H).V:* 94, 15–17.   [40] *CA I.1. CMG (H).V:* 90, 25.
[41] *SD I.6. CMG (H).III:* 42, 31–2; 43, 1.
[42] It is problematic to interpret what exactly Aretaeus meant by *hypochondria*. The heart, the lungs, the liver or the diaphragm can be considered as being below the ribs, depending on the position of the body and its relation to the observer. Actually, all these organs are also mentioned during the discussion of *melancholia* along with the term *hypochondria* (*SD I.5. CMG (H).III*). Perhaps it is another word for innards, like *splachna*, which had been vaguely and fluidly used by the ancient authors as mind-words (Padel, 1994: 26).
[43] *CA I.1. CMG (H).V:* 92, 27–8.   [44] *CA I.1. CMG (H).V:* 96, 19–21; 24–5.
[45] The latter are the specific places where Erasistratus (the *dura mater*) and Herophilus (the fourth ventricle) had placed the ruling principle (Rocca 2003: 37–8).

49

head is the site of perception and the starting point of the nerves'; *CA I.1. CMG (H).V*: 92, 28–9).[46]

This wide dispersion of body parts – which can remind us of the Hippocratic innards – reflects the way in which the author dealt with conflicting sources. His lax eclecticism allowed him to allocate the disease to different parts of the body throughout various explanations without the need to explain the contradictions. Apparently, when facing the crucial question about where the mind resides (hence, where delirium occurs), Celsus – faithful to his 'middle way'– had avoided committing to any specific organ, whereas Aretaeus seems to be suggesting that it is mainly located in the head and nerves, but several other parts can also be involved. In this way, it could be argued that unlike Celsus, Aretaeus did embrace the dichotomous encephalo- versus cardiocentric dispute. This is especially evident when he opposes an affection of the head and the nerves (*phrenitis*) to conditions with altered emotions, behaviours and thinking, which originate in the thoracic organs (ἐν τοῖσι σπλάγχνοισι, *SD I.6. CMG (H).III.6*: 42, 31) – particularly in the heart (*mania–melancholia*). Of course, this scheme is far from perfect, and there are several instances where he contradicts this pattern. Nevertheless, his lax eclecticism enables him to incorporate these apparent contradictions without feeling the need to justify anything.

The discussion about pathophysiological mechanisms is also illustrative of lax eclecticism in action. Very schematically, a number of fixed solid organs (discussed above) and a few fluids and moving entities (humours,[47] *pneuma* and heat) are used to elucidate the workings of the mind, of consciousness and their impairment.[48] These elements are alternately involved, and

[46] A similar idea is easily deducible from the extant fragments by Erasistratus (Rocca 2003: 37–9). In the case of Herophilus, a certain connection seems to have been implied, although the exact relationship between nerves, perceptions and what we now designate as the fourth ventricle is less clearly understood (von Staden 1989: 254).

[47] Beyond the explicit allusions to Hippocrates and the use of Ionic language, these humoural ideas – which are ubiquitous throughout the treatise – reinforce the above-mentioned hypothesis that Aretaeus could be considered as a non-sectarian author who claimed Hippocratic authority. Indeed, probably based on the impact of *On the nature of man*, humoural explanations were regarded as a defining feature of Hippocratic followers from Alexandrian medicine onwards (Nutton 2008: 90).

[48] Some scholars (including McDonald, 2009a: 91, 96) have remarked that the emphasis in Aretaeus' nosography lies on the primary qualities rather than the humours themselves.

different theories can be used to justify different findings and treatments regardless of their intrinsic contradictions.

The source of the *phrenitic* symptoms is τὸ πνεῦμα ξηρόν τε καὶ λεπτὸν ἐόν ('the dry and thin *pneuma*').[49] Therefore, the tension (*tonos*) of this *pneuma* becomes relevant for the treatment: if *phrenitis* has turned into *syncope* and the patient faints, the only cure is wine[50] because 'it adds *tonos* to the *tonos* and awakens the benumbed *pneuma*'.[51] In this example the *pneuma* provides certain capacities and is clearly more than a mere vapour. Inevitably this shares a family resemblance to Stoic ideas about the *pneuma*. However, later on it is a 'hot and dry breathing' that causes delirium,[52] along with the 'innate heat' (*oikeiou thalpeos*).[53] The author is offering similar though not strictly identical ideas such as *anapnoê* and *pneuma*, or *thermê* and *thalpeos*. There is neither internal nor external evidence to be sure whether they refer to the same phenomenon. As a result, we can either hypothesise that Aretaeus was eclectically drawing his theoretical explanations from diverse sources, or that he was using the terminology in a *sumphoretic* manner. In any case, it is relevant to highlight that according to his view, some form of heat and some airy matter as well as dryness were at the centre of the problem (and also of the solution, because by adding tension to the airy matter through wine the symptoms allegedly subsided).

When trying to find further correlations between symptoms, mechanisms and treatment, we should bear in mind that impaired perceptions were the core problem in *phrenitic* patients according to Aretaeus, and that they triggered delirium. According to the previous explanations, this delirium was caused by a hot and dry airy matter. Thus, it is not surprising that the treatment needs to

---

Through this emphasis such scholars aim at supporting the idea that Aretaeus belonged to the Pneumatic sect, and they base their case on the description of the tenets of Pneumatic medicine offered by Verbecke (1945: 91). The reasoning, however, seems a circular one, for Verbecke has used Aretaeus' text to define some of the characteristics of Pneumatism.

[49] *CA I. CMG (H).V.I*: 94, 23.

[50] Note that contrary to the Hippocratic sources, wine has now become an acceptable treatment.

[51] τόνῳ δὲ προσθεῖναι τόνον, καὶ πνεῦμα νεναρκωμένον ἐγεῖραι (*CA I. CMG (H).V.I*: 97, 25).

[52] ἀναπνοὴ θερμή τε καὶ ξηρή (*CA I. CMG (H).V.I*: 96, 26).

[53] οἰκείου θάλπεος (*CA I. CMG (H).V.I*: 96, 29).

succeed at τὸ μὲν ξηρὸν ἀμβλύνεται ('blunting the dryness'),[54] which allows that καθαρεύεται δὲ τῆς ὀμίχλης ἡ αἴσθησις ('the senses become purified from the mist'),[55] which, in turn, cures the patient.

On the other hand, however, this dryness, which seems to cause delirium by compromising the *aisthêsis*, produces the exact opposite effect in patients with *kausôn*, that is, above-normal perception:

ἐξήρανται γὰρ τἆλλα … αἴσθησις ξύμπασα καθαρή, διάνοια λεπτή, γνώμη μαντική … ἐπεὶ δὲ τάδε ἐξήντλησε ἡ νοῦσος, καὶ ἀπὸ τῶν ὀφθαλμῶν τὴν ἀχλὺν ἔλε, ὁρέουσι τά τε ἐν τῷ ἠέρι. *SA II.4. CMG (H). II*: 23, 28; 24, 2–3; 10–11.

The other [organs] dry up … the *aisthêsis* is absolutely pure, the *dianoia* subtle, and the *gnômê* prophetic … Once the disease has drained it [the wetness] off, and has lifted the mist from the eyes, they can see what there is in the air.[56]

The mist metaphor is also used in another passage, which contradicts yet again the previous two.[57] We have mentioned that post-Hellenistic medicine considered *phrenitis* to be a wakeful disease that could be treated with sleep-inducing remedies. Accordingly, Aretaeus considers that the treatment to achieve sleep ὀμίχλην τῆσι αἰσθήσεσι παρέχει: βαρὺ δὲ καὶ νωθὲς ὀμίχλη, ἥπερ ὕπνου ἀρχή ('brings about mist to the *aisthêsis*; a heavy and dulling mist, which is the origin of sleep').[58]

In a nutshell Aretaeus has told us that dryness causes a mist that dulls perceptions in *phrenitis*, dryness can enable above-normal perception in *kausôn* by lifting the mist from the eyes and finally sleep cures *phrenitis* by bringing about mist to the *aisthêsis*. These inconsistencies are another testimony of lax eclecticism, of the

---

[54] *CA I. CMG (H).V.1*: 98, 5.　　[55] *CA I. CMG (H).V.1*: 98, 5.

[56] Oberhelman (1993: 960) recognises in this passage the Poseidonian ideas that the soul of the dying is capable of prediction. Galen, on the other hand, mentions in *QAM* (*Teubner 4*: 42–3) that the association of extreme dryness with intelligence is of Platonic origin. Regardless of whether this is a forced Galenic interpretation or not, it is likely that there was some ongoing discussion about the influence of dryness on the soul. In this way, this passage could be a synthetic effort by Aretaeus to make such diverse traditions compatible.

[57] The mist metaphor reminds us of Galen's smoke that travels to the eyes causing hallucinations, which suggests that similar images were regularly used to explain such phenomena.

[58] *CA I. CMG (H).V.1*: 94, 23–4.

syncretic usage of sources and of a flexible understanding of the primary qualities. (The contradiction could also evidence an important weakness in such a theory, which needed to explain all the available pathologies through a reduced number of possible combinations of qualities.)

On the other end of the spectrum, 'innate coldness' (*psuxis emphutos*) – an antonym of the *phrenitic oikeiou thalpeos*, bearing in mind Aretaeus' lax use of terminology[59] – was the cause of the opposite condition, namely, *lethargy*.[60] As a matter of fact, the emphasis on the coldness of *lethargy* as opposed to the heat of *phrenitis* is possibly the reason why Aretaeus did not consider fever to be part of this condition (unlike Celsus and other post-Hellenistic works). However, such an omission reveals a case of syncretism when addressing the treatment:

τέγξιες τῆς κεφαλῆς, αἵπερ καὶ τοῖσι φρενιτικοῖσι. ἀμφοῖν γὰρ αἱ αἰσθήσιες πλέαι γίγνονται ἀτμῶν, ἃς ἀπελαύνειν χρὴ ψύξεϊ καὶ στύψει, ῥοδίνου καὶ κισσοῦ χυλῷ, ἢ ἐξατμίζειν ἐς διαπνοὴν τοῖσι λεπτύνουσι... *CA I.2. CMG (H). V:* 99, 11–13.

Moistening of the head exactly like amongst *phrenitics*. In both [in *phrenitis* and *lethargy*] perceptions become full of vapours, which we need to drive out through chilling and condensing with juices made of roses and ivy, or evaporate them in transpiration through thinning treatments...

In other words, although this treatment seems to be targeting the pathophysiological mechanism in the case of *phrenitis*, the author is recommending moistening and cooling a patient affected by a moist and cold disease in the case of *lethargy*. In all probability, Aretaeus was transmitting remedies accepted by the tradition (as becomes evident when contrasting the passage with the *Anonymus Parisinus, II.3 1–6*: 14, 16). Remarkable, though, is the fact that his lax eclecticism admitted such evident contradictions.

---

[59] If these concepts are in any way related to the Aristotelian notion of *emphutos thermotês* ('innate heat'), we have another faint 'family resemblance' with a different school of thought. Annas pointed out (1994: 17–20) that the concept of innate heat and its relation to the soul and to the *pneuma* can be traced back to Aristotle. In any case, the link would be with the concept itself, but not with the specificities of the theory, because Aristotle considered *lethargy* to be caused by excessive moist and heat.

[60] ληθαργικοῖσι ... ψῦξις γὰρ ἔμφυτος ἡ αἰτίη ('for lethargics ... innate cold is the cause', *CA I.2. CMG (H). V:* 98, 9).

This passage could also be hinting at another opposition between *lethargy* and *phrenitis*: we have discussed the dry and thin *pneuma* involved in the aetiology of the latter. Perhaps the *atmoi* that need to be cleansed are equivalent to *pneuma*? Be that as it may, there are yet other airy matters involved: *phusas*. '*Lethargy* causes a confluence of gas both in the abdomen and the whole body, through inactivity, lassitude and swoon. They need to be exhaled by movement and wakefulness'.[61] In summary, in both opposing conditions Aretaeus is involving different forms of airy matter (referred to with various terms) that affect consciousness and perceptions, which are somehow related to breathing and need to be removed through treatment.[62]

Notwithstanding these examples of lack of coherence, it is of note that perceptions are often at the centre of most explanations of phenomena related to consciousness, and there is an explicit attempt to target the pathophysiological mechanism with the treatment, in order to cure the condition. On other occasions, however, it was not the bodily processes causing disease that Aretaeus targeted, but the *locus affectus*. In *lethargy*, apart from the gassy abdomen, the compromise of head and nerves justified the treatment with castoreum.[63]

ἐκ προσαγωγῆς δὲ τὸ καστόριον ἀλεαίνει· κεφαλῆσι δὲ καὶ ἄλλως ξύμφορον, ὅτιπερ τὰ νεῦρα πάντη ἐνθένδε περιφύεται· νούσων δὲ νεύρων καστόριον ἰητήριον. *CA I.2. CMG (H).V*: 100, 38–9; 101, 1.

Castoreum makes them [the head and the *aisthêsis*] warm in a gradual manner. It is also otherwise useful for the head, precisely because from all around it the nerves originate, and castoreum is the cure for diseases of the nerves.

---

[61] φυσέων γὰρ ξυναγωγὸν λήθαργος καὶ ἐν τῆσι κοιλίησι καὶ ἐν τῷ ὅλῳ σκήνεϊ ἀργίη καὶ νωθίη καὶ ἀψυχίη· διαπνευστικὸν δὲ κίνησις ἠδὲ ἐγρήγορσις (*CA I.2. CMG (H).V*: 100, 4–6).

[62] As I have remarked in relation to the organs affected, this vague assimilation of *pneuma*, *atmoi* and *phusas* has echoes with the innards as the elements that enabled consciousness according to the tragic poets. Padel (1994: 51) has pointed out that wind, breath in the world and breath in human beings are related to intellectual activity in some pre-Socratic philosophers.

[63] *Castoreum* refers to the strong-smelling secretion of beavers, which was broadly used as a remedy during antiquity and the Middle Ages (Hünermörder C. in 'Beaver' Brill's New Pauly online, https://referenceworks.brill.com/display/entries/NPOE/e216710 .xml?rskey=H5mNx1&result=1 (last accessed April 2025)).

This compound illustrates very eloquently the way in which post-Hellenistic medical writers worked, and how extended the 'pharmaceuticalisation' of excessive sleep was. There must have been a powerful tradition of treating *lethargy* with castoreum; hence, each author justified its use through his particular understanding of the condition. Unlike Aretaeus, who based his justification in the *locus affectus*, other authors based it in the symptoms. Thus, Celsus emphasises its stimulating effects (*Med. 3.19*: 2), similar to the author of the *Anonymus Parisinus*, who also considered its awakening faculty (*Anon. Paris. II.3, 7*: 16, 16).

Finally, many other therapeutic recommendations in Aretaeus targeted specific symptoms and aimed at counteracting them without any evident consideration of the pathophysiological mechanisms involved. As seen in *On medicine*, most of them are described specifically for the treatment of *phrenitis*.[64] We can find the use of conversation (again therapy through the spoken word): non-upsetting words by visitors are advised (*CA I. CMG (H).V.1*: 92, 1–2). Also, a similar conclusion to Celsus is drawn regarding the debate about light–darkness: either choice should be based on the reaction – in each particular patient – to brightness or shadows; whichever triggers 'false' or 'alien images' should be avoided (*CA I. CMG (H).V.1*: 92, 2–7).

These coincidences, again, point towards debates that were likely taking place in his day. Aretaeus' singularity is that, thanks to his lax eclecticism, he was able to combine *phrenitic*-specific approaches with general therapies for acute diseases, treatments justified by physio-pathological explanations with certain others whose rationale contradicted the previous ones, and yet other therapies – common to several post-Hellenistic sources – without any physiological correlate.

In terms of the notion of illness emerging from the relationship between pathophysiological mechanism and therapy, we could

---

[64] But not all of them. There is an example of a synthetic approach to the sources when the author combines the *phrenitic*-specific therapies with others that are useful for all acute diseases (like the Hippocratic examples): ἐπεὶ δὲ καὶ θώρηκα ἐν πάσῃσι τῇσι ὀξείῃσι νούσοισι ἀκέεσθαι χρή ... ἐπὶ δὲ τοῖσι φρενιτικοῖσι καὶ μάλα χρὴ τάδε μειλίσσειν ('given that in all acute diseases the thorax needs to be healed ... in *phrenitic* patients it is particularly necessary to sweeten all these [organs]', *CA I. CMG (H).V.1*: 96, 19–20; 25–6).

claim that Aretaeus' position was intermediate between Celsus and Galen. On the one hand, as in Celsus, several treatments are aimed at specific symptoms regardless of the underlying mechanisms of disease; on the other, when Aretaeus advises targeting the mist or the dryness that compromises perceptions and the *tonos*, we can see a link between therapy and mechanism, which will be more developed in Galen. In any case, he is clearly distanced from the Hippocratic medical writers in the sense that diseases are conceived as individual nosological entities, where the links between clinical features, localisations, mechanisms and treatments are stronger.

In summary, we can see that an important aspect of the post-Hellenistic descriptions of wakeful impaired consciousness is to separate delirium, which was already well known to the Hippocratic doctors, from some more recently described diseases through a taxonomical system of oppositions. Some of these novel conditions, such as *melancholia* and *mania*, would be nowadays classified as mental illness; others, *lethargy* and *cardiacum*, could be subsumed in our idea of impaired consciousness, for they correspond to drowsy and total loss of consciousness, respectively; and yet others remind us of neurological disorders, such as dementia. Naturally, in this context – more constrained by the nosological classification – there is a stronger sense of unity in the notion of disease (particularly in the link between symptoms and treatments) than what we had seen among the Hippocratic authors.

CHAPTER 5

GALEN'S DELIRIUM: HOT AND DRY *DUSKRASIA* OF THE *HÊGEMONIKON*

As stated in Chapter 1, Galen's system was centred in the intersection between an anatomical axis, which determined the site to which the treatment needed to be applied, and a humoural-physiological axis that guided the quality that needed to be allopathically counterbalanced, as well as the quantity of the correction required. This shift of focus, from the Hippocratic emphasis on clinical descriptions, and the post-Hellenistic stress on nosologic taxonomy, conditioned a different understanding of impaired consciousness and mental illness.[1] Although Galen did not disregard diseases and symptoms, in his approach these elements are subordinated to his main concerns: the organ affected, the type of *duskrasia* and the degree of impairment in the qualities (required by his system to choose an adequate treatment). Such a change of emphasis had powerful consequences, for it often blurred the boundaries between impaired consciousness and madness.

The efforts that we have seen in *On medicine* and in Aretaeus' work (also in the *Introduction* and the *Medical definitions*) to distinguish *phrenitis* from other forms of mental conditions – particularly from *melancholia* and *mania* – will change.

γίνονται μὲν οὖν καὶ μετὰ πυρετοῦ βλάβαι τῶν ἡγεμονικῶν ἐνεργειῶν, ὡς ἐπὶ φρενίτιδός τε καὶ ληθάργου γίνονται δὲ καὶ χωρὶς πυρετοῦ, καθάπερ ἐπὶ μανίας τε καὶ μελαγχολίας· ὥσπερ γε καὶ κατὰ συμπάθειάν τε καὶ πρωτοπάθειαν ἐγκεφάλου· τὰ μὲν ἠκριβωμένα τοῖς ἰδίοις συμπτώμασι καὶ διηνεκῆ καὶ μὴ προηγησαμένων ἑτέρων γενόμενα κατὰ πρωτοπάθειαν τὰ δὲ ... ἐφ᾽ ἑτέροις τε συστάντα κατὰ συμπάθειαν ... *Loc. Aff. 3, 7. K.VIII*: 166, 5–14.

The activities of the *hêgemonikon* ('ruling part') can be damaged sometimes with fever as in *phrenitis* and *lethargy*, and sometimes without fever as in *mania* and *melancholia*. Additionally, the damage to the brain can be *sympathetic* or

---

[1] In this sense I agree with Nutton (2013b: 121), who claims that unlike Aretaeus, Galen is not interested in nosography but in the 'intellectual bases of medical practice, from which his therapeutic flows'.

protopathetic (that is, the primary affection is in the brain). We can accurately detect the latter when the symptoms are characteristic [of the brain], continuous, and are not preceded by symptoms of other parts. The former ... is associated with [symptoms] proceeding from other parts [of the body] through sympathy ...

Although I consider that Galen's approach strongly distances him from his forerunners', this passage suggests that he still engaged in the debate around boundaries between different forms of impaired consciousness (*phrenitis–lethargy*), and the fuzzy edges that separated the former from mental illness (*mania* and *melancholia*). Additionally, the passage highlights how the distinction between chronic and acute diseases, which was a key organising feature in the post-Hellenistic authors to differentiate these conditions, is irrelevant for Galen. The only time-reference included is the continuous nature of the symptoms in primary diseases of the brain.

Actually, Galen's main concern here seems to be the localisation of the disease. It is crucial for him to know whether the damage was produced in the brain or somewhere else in order to decide where to apply the treatment. In a very similar passage from *On the causes of symptoms* he adds:

ὀνομάζονται δε φρενίτιδες μὲν αἱ μετὰ πυρετῶν, μανίαι δὲ αἱ χωρὶς τούτων, ποτὲ μὲν τοῖς δακνώδεσι καὶ θερμοῖς ἑπόμεναι χυμοῖς, ὁποῖος ὁ τῆς ξανθῆς χολῆς ἐστι μάλιστα, πολλάκις δὲ κατὰ τὴν δυσκρασίαν τὴν ἐπὶ τὸ θερμότερον αὐτοῦ τοῦ ἐγκεφάλου συνιστάμεναι μόναι δ' αἱ μελαγχολικαὶ παράνοιαι ψυχρότερον ἔχουσι τὸν αἴτιον χυμόν. *Caus. Symp. 2, 7. K.VII*: 202, 5–11.

[Deliriums, *paraphrosunai*] with fever are called *phrenitis*, whereas [deliriums, *paraphrosunai*] without fever are called *mania*. Sometimes they follow pungent and hot humours, particularly yellow bile; many other times they are associated with a hot *duskrasia* of the brain itself. Only melancholic deliriums (*melancholikai paranoiai*) have a colder humour as a cause.

In this case the aim is to explain the kind of humours involved in each condition. Because both *phrenitis* and *mania* happen in the brain, and are caused by similar kinds of humours, they will very likely receive a similar treatment. As a result, for Galen it is not as important as it was for the other post-Hellenistic doctors to distinguish one from the other, and therefore, he will not put as much effort as they did into trying to expose the difference. As a matter of fact, allusions to *mania* are very scarce in the works under scrutiny.[2] Only the presence or absence of fever is enough to put a label to either condition, which – in all probability – will anyway be treated in a similar manner. On the other hand, *melancholia* is caused by the opposite mixture and therefore will require the opposite treatment. Hence, as we will see later, it is worth distinguishing this condition from the other two.

Going back to the dichotomy *phrenitis–mania*, Galen classifies as the former several conditions that other authors had associated with the latter.

εἰσὶν μὲν γὰρ αὐτῆς ἁπλαῖ μὲν δύο, σύνθετος δὲ ἐξ ἀμφοῖν ἡ τρίτη. τινὲς μὲν γὰρ τῶν φρενιτικῶν, οὐδὲν ὅλως σφαλλόμενοι περὶ τὰς αἰσθητικὰς διαγνώσεις τῶν ὁρατῶν, οὐ κατὰ φύσιν ἔχουσι ταῖς διανοητικαῖς κρίσεσιν ἔνιοι δ᾽ ἔμπαλιν ἐν μὲν ταῖς διανοήσεσιν οὐδὲν σφάλλονται, παρατυπωτικῶς δὲ κινοῦνται κατὰ αἰσθήσεις, ἄλλοις δέ τισιν κατ᾽ ἄμφω βεβλάφθαι συμβέβηκεν. *Loc. Aff. 4. 2. K.VIII*: 225, 13–18; 226, 1.

There are two types of it [of *phrenitis*] that are simple and a third type, which is a combination of both. Some *phrenitic* patients are not at all mistaken about the perceptual distinction (*aisthêtikas diagnôseis*) of what they see, but their intellectual judgement (*dianoêtikais krisesin*) is not normal. Others, on the contrary, do not suffer from intellectual errors but their perceptions are misrepresented (*paratupôtikôs*). In yet certain others both damages are combined.

The extreme types are illustrated by a corresponding example: the first one involves a patient whose perceptions were sound enough to recognise the objects that he threw through the window, but whose judgement did not allow him to acknowledge the senselessness and danger of what he was doing. For the second kind the author uses his own experience with *phrenitis*, when he started to have visual hallucinations but was still intellectually sound enough to tell his friends what to do to cure him of the disease. The similarities between these two typologies of *phrenitis*, and the other authors' contrasts between *mania* and *phrenitis*, respectively, are not difficult to spot, particularly if we apply the analysis of connectedness and alertness that was used in Aretaeus (indeed the first variety of Galenic *phrenitis* is conceptually

---

[2] Clarke and Rose (2013: 59) have also remarked that Galen's allusions to *mania* are 'brief and superficial'.

equivalent to Aretaeus' definition of *mania* in *SD I.6. CMG (H). III*: 43, 1–4).[3] Clearly, Galen was not particularly interested in clinically distinguishing two diseases that required the same treatment, even if he was able to clinically differentiate the diverse nature of the symptoms.

On the other hand, in diseases that warranted an alternative therapeutic approach due to their different pathophysiology or bodily localisation, the distinct clinical presentations are more explicitly stated. Such are the cases of *melancholia* and various conditions with fever. In the case of *melancholia*, there is a thorough description of the kind of mental disturbance that one should expect.

οἱ φόβοι συνεδρεύουσι τοῖς μελαγχολικοῖς, οὐκ ἀεὶ δὲ ταὐτὸν εἶδος τῶν παρὰ φύσιν αὐτοῖς γίγνεται φαντασιῶν, εἴγε ὁ μέν τις ὀστρακοῦς ᾤετο γεγονέναι καὶ διὰ τοῦτ' ἐξίστατο τοῖς ἀπαντῶσιν, ὅπως μὴ συντριβείη θεώμενος δέ τις ἄλλος ἀλεκτρυόνας ᾄδοντας ὥσπερ ἐκεῖνοι τὰς πτέρυγας προσέκρουον πρὸ ᾠδῆς, οὕτω καὶ αὐτὸς τοὺς βραχίονας προσκρούων ταῖς πλευραῖς ἐμιμεῖτο τὴν φωνὴν τῶν ζῴων. φόβος δ' ἦν ἄλλῳ, μή πως ὁ βαστάζων τὸν κόσμον Ἄτλας ἀποσείσηται κεκμηκὼς αὐτόν, οὕτως τε καὶ αὐτὸς συντριβείη καὶ ἡμᾶς αὐτῷ συναπολέσειεν· ... διαφέρονται δὲ ἀλλήλων οἱ μελαγχολικοί, τὸ μὲν φοβεῖσθαι καὶ δυσθυμεῖν καὶ μέμφεσθαι τῇ ζωῇ καὶ μισεῖν τοὺς ἀνθρώπους ἅπαντες ἔχοντες, ἀποθανεῖν δ' ἐπιθυμοῦντες οὐ πάντες, ἀλλ' ἔστιν ἐνίοις αὐτῶν αὐτὸ δὴ τοῦτο κεφάλαιον τῆς μελαγχολίας, τὸ περὶ τοῦ θανάτου δέος ... *Loc. Aff. 3.10. K.VIII*: 190, 1–15.

Fears accompany *melancholic* patients, but the type of abnormal apparitions is not always the same: someone believed that he had become a pot and therefore he warded off everybody to avoid being crushed; another one, after hearing a cock crow and observing how it flapped its wings before crowing, imitated the voice of the animal and beat his arms against his sides. Somebody else was afraid that Atlas, who bears the [weight of the] universe, might somehow shake out of exhaustion, thereby destroying himself and killing us all ... *Melancholic* patients differ from one another; all of them have fears, are despondent about their lives, dissatisfied, and hate mankind, but not all of them want to die. There are some whose main *melancholic* feature is the fear of death ...

Naturally, if *mania*, *phrenitis* and *melancholia* all occur in the brain, and they all involve hallucinations or impaired judgement, but the former two are caused by hot and dry humours, whereas the

---

[3] And also Celsus' third type of *insania*, where patients suffered from chronic delusions like Ajax and Orestes or became foolish in their *animus*, but were not deceived in their *mens* by *vanas imagines*.

latter is due to cold and moist ones, it is crucial to differentiate them, for they will have opposite treatments. This might be the reason why Galen's description of *melancholia* is so thorough, while beyond the fever, *mania* and *phrenitis* are barely distinguished. Concerning the specific symptoms, it is interesting to highlight that – like with Aretaeus – the kind of mental disturbances that Galen is describing would be now considered as delusions rather than hallucinations or delirium, for they seem to be structured, stable in time, and apparently, reasoning is not affected (judgement is). Furthermore, the story about the man who believed himself to be a pot and was afraid of being crushed reminds us of Aretaeus' patient who thought he had become a brick and avoided water, for fear of dissolving.

Apart from *melancholia*, the other diseases that could be easily confused with *phrenitis* – and therefore needed to be more accurately distinguished – were several other conditions with fever and delirium, which did not originate in the brain.

παραφροσύναι μὲν οὖν γίγνονται κἀπὶ τῷ τῆς γαστρὸς στόματι κακοπραγοῦντι καὶ διακαέσι πυρετοῖς καὶ πλευρίτισιν καὶ περιπνευμονίαις· ἀλλ' αἱ διὰ τὰς φρένας ἐγγὺς τῶν φρενιτικῶν εἰσιν· ἐπὶ μὲν γὰρ τοῖς ἄλλοις μορίοις πάσχουσι καὶ τοῖς διακαέσι πυρετοῖς ἐν ταῖς παρακμαῖς αὐτῶν ἡ παραφροσύνη καθίσταται· ταῖς φρενίτισι δ' ἴδιον ἐξαίρετον ὑπάρχει τὸ μηδ' ἐν ταῖς παρακμαῖς τῶν πυρετῶν παύεσθαι τὴν παραφροσύνην· οὐ γὰρ ἐπὶ συμπαθείᾳ κατ' ἐκείνην τὴν νόσον ὁ ἐγκέφαλος πάσχει, ἀλλὰ κατ' ἰδιοπάθειάν τε καὶ πρωτοπάθειαν κάμνει, καὶ διὰ τοῦτο κατὰ βραχύ τε συνίσταται τοῦτο τὸ πάθος καὶ οὐκ ἐξαίφνης παρακόπτουσιν ἢ ἀθρόως ... οὐκ ὀλίγα τε συμπτώματα προηγεῖται τῆς κατασκευῆς αὐτοῦ, καὶ καλεῖται γε πάντα ταῦτα φρενιτικὰ σημεῖα...

... μέγα μὲν γὰρ καὶ διὰ πολλοῦ χρόνου τὸ πνεῦμα τοῖς ἐπ' ἐγκεφάλῳ φρενιτικοῖς ἐφεξῆς ἐστιν ἀεί· τοῖς δ' ἐπὶ ταῖς φρεσὶν ἀνώμαλον, ὡς καὶ μικρόν ποτε γενέσθαι, καὶ πυκνόν, αὖθίς τέ ποτε μέγα καὶ στεναγματῶδες. *Loc. Aff. 5.4. K.VIII:* 329, 5–19; 331, 15–18.

Deliriums also occur in dysfunctions of the mouth of the stomach, ardent fevers, *pleuritis* and *peripneumonias*. Those that originate in the diaphragm are nearly *phrenitic*. Whereas in affections of other parts and ardent fevers, delirium declines during the abatement of the disease, it is singular and characteristic in *phrenitis* that delirium does not cease when the fever is descending. Indeed, in such a disease [*phrenitis*] the brain is not affected through sympathy but suffers primarily by itself. This is the reason why this disease progresses slowly and frenzy neither appears suddenly nor immediately ... Not a few symptoms precede this condition, and they are all called *phrenitic* signs...

... Breathing in *phrenitics* of the brain is always deep and with intervals between one another; in [*phrenitics*] of the diaphragm, conversely, [breathing] is uneven: sometimes superficial and frequent, sometimes deep and like sighs.

Galen's clinical description in these passages is thorough. He goes through all the *phrenitic* symptoms,[4] which mostly coincide with the descriptions of the disease that we have found in the other surviving post-Hellenistic medical writers. The nuance comes in Galen's practical approach. As stated above, he only goes to great lengths to distinguish between conditions whenever such a distinction impacts on the treatment. In this case, the *locus affectus* is at stake: by being able to tell *phrenitis* from *pleuritis*, *peripneumonia* or 'diaphragmatic near-*phrenitis*', he will know the correct part of the body to which the treatment needs to be applied.

Finally, this focus on anatomical location and physiologic mechanism is even more evident when Galen contrasts *phrenitis* with drowsy impaired consciousness (*lethargy*), because they were construed as perfectly opposite conditions in terms of symptoms, humours and qualities involved. Actually, they are conceived as the two prototypical extremes of a spectrum, in the middle of which one can find a mixture of both (which is designated by some authors as *tuphomania*).[5] Its characterisation is the only example that reminds us of the Hippocratic description of vigil coma:

invenies enim multos freneticos <nec> surgentes omnino nec elevare potentes oculos, sed in eodem loco manentes similiter letargicis. *Comm. Hip. 2. CMG*: 188, 15–17. *K.VII*: 655.

You will find many *phrenitic* patients who cannot get up at all, nor open their eyes. Instead, they remain in the same place, like *lethargics* do.[6]

So far, we can suggest that, on the one hand, Galen's system obscured the distinction between impaired consciousness and

---

[4] McDonald (2009a: 128–39) offers an in-depth analysis of all the symptoms throughout Galen's corpus.

[5] As Devinant (2020: 196) points out, Galen refuses to talk about *tuphomania*. Instead he considers it as two concomitant diseases, namely, *phrenitis* and *lethargy*.

[6] Unlike the Hippocratic examples these patients keep their eyes shut. Nevertheless, the fact that Galen considers them to be suffering from *phrenitis* suggests that they were not in an actual coma.

a specific form of mental illness (*mania*), which had reached a rather sophisticated degree of characterisation during the post-Hellenistic period. On the other, it preserved clear boundaries between *phrenitis* and certain conditions that – according to his system – required different therapeutic approaches (*melancholia* and *lethargy*). The subordination of every finding to his tripartite theoretical framework becomes even more evident when trying to independently explore the different components of the notion of disease that we have been chasing in the other sources. The system is so closely knit that it is virtually impossible to isolate each element: we cannot choose to only explore symptoms, or affected organs, or mechanisms or treatments without mentioning the other three.

Galen's notion of disease: the perfect meshing of symptoms, *loci affecti*, mechanisms and treatments

Undoubtedly, hallucinations still constitute an important element of *phrenitis*: ἀγρυπνίας ἢ καὶ τινας ὕπνους θορυβώδεις ἐπὶ φαντάσμασιν ἐναργέσιν, ὡς καὶ κράξαι ποτὲ καὶ ἀναπηδῆσαι ('insomnia, or some turbulent dreams with such vivid apparitions that [affected individuals] sometimes scream and jump up from bed').[7] However, there is a coherent theoretical framework that underpins the strong links between such a symptom (abnormal perceptions), a certain part of the body and the mechanism that explains it.

ὅτ' ἂν γὰρ ἀθροισθῇ τις ἐν ἐγκεφάλῳ χολώδης χυμὸς ἅμα πυρετῷ διακαεῖ, παραπλήσιόν τι πάσχει τοῖς ὑπὸ πυρὸς ὀπτωμένοις, καὶ κατὰ τοῦτο λιγνύν τινα γεννᾷν πέφυκεν ... ἥτις λιγνὺς συνδιεκπίπτουσα τοῖς ἐπὶ τὸν ὀφθαλμὸν ἀφικνουμένοις ἀγγείοις, αἰτία γίνεται τῶν φαντασμάτων αὐτοῖς. *Loc. Aff. 4.2. K. VIII*: 227, 15–18; 228, 1–2.

When a certain bilious humour accumulates in the brain accompanied by fever it overheats, resembling something being roasted by fire, from which some smoke comes out ... This smoke, flowing through into vessels that arrive in the eyes, becomes the cause of their apparitions.

[7] *Loc. Aff. 5.4. K.VIII*: 330, 1–3.

63

This passage relates the abnormal perceptions to a primary problem in the brain, a secondary problem in the eyes and a mechanism involving humours. Furthermore, Galen elsewhere clarifies that

καὶ τοίνυν αἱ βλάβαι τῶν αἰσθητικῶν ἐνεργειῶν κοιναὶ μὲν ἁπασῶν ἀναισθησίαι τινές εἰσιν, ἢ δυσαισθησίαι ... καὶ πρὸς τούτοις ἔτι δύο ἐξαίρετα, τὸ μὲν ἀγρυπνία, τὸ δὲ κῶμα ... ἐφεξῆς δ᾽ ἂν εἴη τὰς τῶν ἡγεμονικῶν ἐνεργειῶν βλάβας διελθεῖν, καὶ πρώτης γε τῆς φανταστικῆς. ἔστι δὲ καὶ ταύτης ... ὃ δὲ κάρος καὶ κατάληψις ... παραφροσύνη ... τὸ δὲ οἷον ἐλλιπὴς καὶ ἄτονος [κίνησις], ὡς ἐν κώμασί τε καὶ ληθάργοις... Symp. Diff. 3.2 CMG (G): 56, 11–12. K.VII: 56; 3.6. CMG (G): 220, 23; 221, 1. K.VII: 58; 3.9. CMG (G): 224, 9–13. K.VII: 60.

The damages common to all the perceptual activities are certain *anaesthesiai* or *dusaesthesiai* ... apart from these, there are also two special ones: sleeplessness and *kôma* ... Subsequently, the damages to the *hêgemonikon* [itself] should be discussed, and firstly those that affect the imagination (*phantastikon*). Amongst them are ... torpor (*karos*) and *catalepsy*, ... delirium (*paraphrosunê*) ... [and] something akin to a defective [movement] lacking tone, as in *kômas* and lethargies ...

In a nutshell, *paraphrosunê* (which invariably presents hallucinations) is associated with a primary dysfunction of the *phantastikon*, dependent on the *hêgemonikon*. It is in the seat of this ruling part of the *psuchê* (the brain) that the problem is generated, and from there it travels to the eyes – the visual organ of the *aisthêtikon*. In other words, according to Galen hallucinations are generated in the brain, and impaired perceptions are a consequence of this phenomenon.

Regarding the other symptom associated with delirium in the HC – speech disturbances – the waning tendency that we have remarked among post-Hellenistic authors persists in Galen. One of the very few occasions where it appears unequivocally associated with a state of impaired consciousness is the intermediate state between *phrenitis* and *lethargy*.

εἰ πυνθάνοιό τι καὶ εἰ διαλέγεσθαι βιάζοιο, δυσχερεῖς ἀποκρίνασθαι καὶ ἀργοί, τὰ πολλὰ δὲ παραφόρως φθεγγόμενοι καὶ οὐκ ὀρθῶς ἀποκρινόμενοι καὶ ληροῦντες εἰκῇ. *Caus. Puls. 4.15. K.IX*: 188, 10–12.

If something is asked of them or they are forced to speak, they will answer slowly and with difficulty. Most times they will mumble deliriously, will not reply correctly and chat randomly.

Because Galen's theoretical framework is so consistent, we have already discussed several examples where the *locus affectus* plays a defining role in the definition of disease. What I would like to emphasise now is how – through his particular approach to this concept – Galen succeeded in coherently integrating most of the organs or affected parts, which had been appearing in the medical tradition since the HC onwards (without resorting to Celsus' uncommitted stance or to Aretaeus' inconsistencies).

Undoubtedly, the primary organ involved in all psychic activities for this author was the brain. Its relevance is revealed in *The art of medicine*: after defining the four *archai* or principles of the body, namely, the brain, the heart, the liver and the testicles (*Ars. Med. CUF 5.2*: 287, 1–2. *K.I:* 319), Galen places the *hêgemonikon* in the brain and associates certain psychic conditions with the impairment in its qualities.

ἡ μέντοι τῶν ἡγεμονικῶν ἐνεργειῶν ἀρετή τε καὶ κακία τῆς ἀρχῆς μόνης ἐστὶν αὐτῆς καθ᾽ ἑαυτὴν γνώρισμα· καλῶ δὲ ἡγεμονικὰς ἐνεργείας τὰς ὑπὸ τῆς ἀρχῆς μόνης γινομένας· ἀγχίνοια μὲν οὖν λεπτομεροῦς οὐσίας ἐγκεφάλου γνώρισμα, βραδυτῆς δὲ διανοίας παχυμεροῦς· εὐμάθεια δ᾽ εὐτυπώτου, καὶ μνήμη μονίμου· ... καὶ τὸ μὲν εὐμετάβολον ἐν δόξαις θερμῆς, τὸ δὲ μόνιμον ψυχρᾶς. *Ars. Med. CUF 6.9*: 290, 11–16; 291, 1–3. *K.I:* 322.

The virtue and defect in the activities of the authoritative part (*hêgemonikon*) are only dependent on the principle (*archê*) in itself. I designate only those [activities] that arise from the *archê* as activities of the *hêgemonikon*. Sagacity (*anchinoia*) is a property of the thin-particled substance of the brain, whereas sluggishness of intellect (*dianoia*) of a dense-particled one; a gift for learning [depends on] a malleable [substance], memory on a stable one; ... and changeability of opinion [is peculiar] to the heat, whereas stability [of opinion] to the cold.

The localisation of the *hêgemonikon* in the brain (*enkephalon*), and its possible alterations as a direct result of the characteristics of its substance (dense–thin, malleable–immalleable, stable–fluid, hot–cold) are explicit.[8] Moreover, there is a surprising degree of sophistication when describing the exact location of the damage:

ἡ δὲ ἀποπληξία διὰ τὴν ἐξαίφνης γένεσιν ἐνδείκνυται ψυχρόν χυμὸν, ἢ παχὺν, ἢ γλίσχρον ἀθρόως πληροῦντα τὰς κυριωτέρας τῶν κατὰ τὸν ἐγκέφαλον κοιλιῶν, οὐ

---

[8] The effects of the qualities of hot and cold on the *hêgemonikon* are in agreement with the theories that we will be discussing. On the other hand, the allusions to a dense or

κατὰ δυσκρασίαν ὅλης τῆς οὐσίας αὐτοῦ γίνεσθαι, καθάπερ ὅ τε λήθαργος καὶ ἡ φρενῖτις, αἵ τε μανίαι καὶ αἱ μελαγχολίαι καὶ αἱ μωρώσεις, ἀπώλειαι τε τῆς μνήμης, ἀμυδρότης τε τῶν αἰσθήσεων, καὶ τῶν κινήσεων ἐκλύσεις. *Loc. Aff. 3.12. K.VIII:* 200, 12–19.

The quick onset of *apoplexy* shows that it originates in a sudden filling of the main cavities in the brain with a cold, dense or viscous humour, and not in a bad mixture (*duskrasia*) of all its [the brain's] substance, which is the case in *lethargy*, *phrenitis*, *mania*, *melancholia* and folly (*môrôsis*), as well as in destructions of memory, faint perceptions and feebleness of movements.

The intersection between the anatomical and the humoural axes is clearly revealed here.[9] Psychic diseases can be differentiated according to the exact location in the brain (the ventricles versus the parenchyma) and the nature and quality of the humour involved.[10]

Other examples illustrate how mapping the *locus affectus* onto the actual body determined where the treatment needed to be applied:

... ἀλλὰ τοῦτό γε τὸ ὀξυρρόδινον ὃ τῇ κεφαλῇ προσφέρομεν ἐπὶ τῶν φρενιτικῶν ... οὐ μόνον τοὺς ἀμεθόδους Θεσσαλείους, ἀλλὰ καὶ τοὺς ἄλλους ἅπαντας ἐξελέγχει φανερῶς, ὅσοι κατὰ τὴν καρδίαν ἡγοῦνται τὸ ψυχῆς ἡγεμονικὸν ὑπάρχειν ... καὶ μὲν δὴ κἀπὶ τῶν ληθαργικῶν οὐδείς ἐστιν ὃς οὐ προσφέρει τῇ κεφαλῇ τὰ βοηθήματα· καὶ τοῦτο γὰρ τὸ πάθος ... γίνεται δ᾽ ἐγκεφάλου πάσχοντος, ἐν ᾧ τῆς ψυχῆς ἐστι τὸ ἡγεμονικόν. *MM XIII.21. LCL:* 400, 7–11; 23–5; 402, 2–3. *K.X:* 928–9.

thin-particled substance have echoes of atomic notions, whereas the malleability (*eutupou*) reminds us of Stoic ideas of *tupôsis*, which – as Pigeaud pointed out – were not alien to Galen (Pigeaud 2008: 573). Interestingly, in *On the elements according to Hippocrates*, Galen states that of all the possible qualities that a substance (*ousia*) might have, it can only be affected by hot, cold, moist and dry, for τῶν γὰρ ἄλλων οὐδὲ μία ποιοτήτων ἀλλοιοῦν οἷα τέ ἐστι τὸ πλησιάζον... ('none of the other qualities [heavy–light; smooth–rough; dense–rarefied; thick–thin] alters whatever is next to them...') (*Elem. Hip. CMG 9:* 130, 15–16. *K.I:* 484). We could interpret by contrasting these passages that certain qualities are more relevant than others.

9 Also evident is the estrangement from the theory of humours as described in *On the nature of man*. The humour remains completely unidentified in this passage and is therefore rather irrelevant. As Devinant (2020: 214) has suggested, its qualities are what really matter.

10 In a later chapter Galen contradicts this principle: the same kind of humours (cold, dense and viscous) are responsible for torpor (*karos*) and epilepsy when affecting the ventricles rather than the 'body of the brain', whereas in *apoplexy* the body is more affected: ... ἐν μὲν τοῖς κάροις τε καὶ ταῖς ἐπιληψίαις αἱ κοιλίαι μὲν μᾶλλον, ἧττον δὲ αὐτὸ τὸ σῶμα τοῦ ἐγκεφάλου πάσχειν εἴωθεν, ἐν δὲ ταῖς ἀποπληξίαις μᾶλλον τὸ σῶμα (*Loc. Aff. 4.3. K.VIII:* 232, 3–6). The only way to make both passages compatible would be to interpret that Galen is referring to relative amounts, that is, in *apoplexy* the affection of the cerebral parenchyma is relatively more important as compared to torpor and epilepsy (even though *apoplexy* still has a predominant affection of the ventricles).

... This *oxyrrhodinum* that we apply to the head of the *phrenitic* patients unquestionably refutes ... not only the amethodical followers of Thessalus, but also all the others who believe that the authoritative part of the *psuchê* (*hêgemonikon*) resides in the heart ... neither is there anybody who would not apply the treatment to the head in *lethargic* patients, for this affection also occurs when the brain, where the *hêgemonikon* of the *psuchê* lies, suffers.

Apart from illustrating Galen's self-advertising technique of discrediting his opponents to highlight his own skills, the passage very clearly shows the way in which his anatomical understanding serves the crucial purpose of providing him with a rationale to guide the treatment of each condition.[11] Furthermore, even the specific location within the brain (for example, the body as opposed to the ventricles, *Loc. Aff. 3.12. K.VIII*: 200, 12–19) can have therapeutic relevance:

διὰ βάθους δὲ κειμένου τοῦ πεπονθότος, ἐπιτεχνᾶσθαι χρὴ τοιοῦτον ἐργάζεσθαι τὸ ὑγιεινόν, ὡς μὴ φθάνειν ἐκλύεσθαι κατὰ τὴν ὁδόν· εἰ μὲν οὖν θερμότερον εἶναι δέοι τοῦ συμμέτρου, μὴ τοσοῦτον μόνον ἔστω θερμότερον, ὅσου δεῖται τὸ πάθος, ἀλλ᾽ ἐξ ἐπιμέτρου προσκείσθω τὸ διὰ τὴν θέσιν ἀναγκαίως προσερχόμενον. *Ars. Med. 28.16*: 364, 7. *K.I*: 384

If the affected part is deeply located, it is necessary to devise [a remedy] to bring about health in such a way that it does not lose its effect prematurely in the passage. Thus, if it needs to be hotter than the normal balance, the heat should not only be increased to the degree that the affection requires, but an extra measure should be added necessarily, in order for it to arrive at the position.

An impressive awareness, indeed, of the pharmacokinetic notion that we currently define as the 'bioavailability' of a drug is shown in this passage. Galen seems to understand – as we currently do – that some fractions of any drug or treatment are lost before they reach the site of action, and therefore, those losses need to be compensated for when calculating the dose. Additionally, there is an unambiguous illustration of the interplay between anatomy and humoural theory. In this sense, I agree with Devinant that *l'humuralisme*

---

[11] The use of *phrenitis* and *lethargy* to prove the encephalic location of the *hêgemonikon* (to the detriment of cardiocentric theories) is a frequent argument. In *On the affected parts* (*Loc. Aff. CMG I.1*: 48, 3–13. *K.VIII*: 19) he uses the same reasoning to disparage Archigenes and his followers, and later on (*Loc. Aff. CMG II.10*: 376, 12–26; 378, 1–3. *K.VIII*: 130–1) he makes with it a *reductio ad absurdum*.

hippocratique is reinterpreted in qualitative terms, but I would also add the quantitative dimension.[12]

The system so far described might appear straightforward and simple: psychic diseases are to be found in the brain, and therefore treated in the head. However, there are nuances. The concept of sympathy (*sympatheia*) complicates the anatomical location of the illnesses.

It is this idea of sympathy that will allow Galen to integrate all the different organs that were considered to be affected in *phrenitis* throughout the tradition. This notion explains how certain conditions that affect different parts of the body (and not primarily the head) can also compromise the *hêgemonikon* and cause psychic disturbances. As Holmes has accurately described, the brain is enmeshed in 'networks crisscrossing the body', thereby making it vulnerable to conditions that originate in distant locations.[13] Several examples of sympathy can be found in *On the affected parts*.

ὅταν μὲν γὰρ ἐκ τῆς κοιλίας ἤτοι γε ἀτμῶν μοχθηρῶν, ἢ καὶ τῶν χυμῶν αὐτῶν ἀναφερομένων ἐπὶ τὸν ἐγκέφαλον, ἡ διάνοια βλάπτηται, πρώτως μὲν οὐκ ἄν τις φαίη πάσχειν τὸν ἐγκέφαλον, οὐ μὴν οὐδ' ἀπαθῆ γε παντάπασιν ὑπάρχειν, ἀλλ' ὅ τι περ ὑπ' αὐτῶν ἐκείνων ὁμολογεῖται, διὰ τοῦ συμπάσχειν ῥήματος ἀληθέστατόν ἐστιν. *Loc. Aff.* CMG I.6: 282, 9–13. *K.VIII*: 48–9.

Whenever deleterious vapours from the bowels or some of the humours in them move up to the brain, intelligence (*dianoia*) is damaged. Nobody would say that the brain is primarily suffering, neither could one claim that it remains completely unharmed. Everybody [all the doctors] agrees that the clearest [way to express it] is through the verb 'sympathise' (*sumpaschein*) [that is, suffers together].

This passage supports Devinant's remark that Galen went one step further than Archigenes: not only did he diagnose the *locus affectus*, not only did he suggest a sympathetic link between the organs, but he also described the mechanism that drove the problem from one organ to the other.[14] The practical importance of the whole explanation is, again, to establish where the treatment should be applied. In this respect, Galen offers one of his several

---

[12] Devinant (2020: 214–5).   [13] Holmes (2013: 150).
[14] Devinant (2020: 251–2). This author describes three stages in the analysis of the *locus affectus* when incorporating the notion of sympathy (235–51).

Galen's notion of disease

self-aggrandising anecdotes. He tells the story of a young man
who had fallen from a certain height and hit his upper back. The
patient developed speechlessness and paralysis in both legs, which
other unskilled doctors were trying to treat:

βουλομένων οὖν τῶν ἰατρῶν ἐνοχλεῖν εἰκῇ, τοῖς μὲν σκέλεσι, διότι παρεῖτο, τῷ δὲ
λάρυγγι διὰ τὸ τῆς φωνῆς πάθημα, κωλύσας ἐγώ, μόνου προενοησάμην τοῦ
πεπονθότος τόπου, καὶ γενομένου ἀφλεγμάντου τοῦ νωτιαίου μετὰ τὴν ἑβδόμην
ἡμέραν ἐπανῆλθεν ἥ τε φωνὴ καὶ τῶν σκελῶν κίνησις τῷ νεανίσκῳ. *Loc. Aff.* CMG
I.6: 284, 19–21; 286, 1–2. *K.VIII*: 51.

I stopped the doctors who wanted to pester him purposelessly in his legs because
of the immobility, and in the larynx due to the affection of the voice, and took care
of the affected part. Once the inflammation in the spinal cord disappeared after
the seventh day, the youth recovered both the voice and the movement in his legs.

Beyond the marketing purposes, the story illustrates how the *locus
affectus* is not always obvious, and the extent to which it is key in
order to provide an effective cure. Other examples of sympathetic
versus protopathetic delirium were presented above, where Galen
explains how to distinguish *pleuritis*, *peripneumonia* and diaphragmatic near-*phrenitis* from actual *phrenitis* (*Loc. Aff. 5.4. K.
VIII*: 329, 5–19; 331, 15–18). All of them illustrate how he was
able to embrace the long tradition of organs affected by *phrenitis*
without renouncing his encephalocentric position.

As exemplified throughout this section, allusions to pathophysiological mechanisms are ubiquitous in most Galenic discussions about symptoms and affected organs. I would now like to
place the focus on therapies, in order to show how all four elements articulate in an integral and rational notion of disease. Galen's
construction of impaired consciousness as a spectrum that ranges
between hot and cold offers a good starting point to illustrate the
above: ἀγρυπνητικαὶ μὲν αἱ ἐγκαύσεις, καταφορικαὶ δ᾽ αἱ ψύξεις
γινόμεναι ('heat triggers insomnia, whereas coldness triggers
drowsiness (*kataphora*)').[15] Naturally, the treatment is aimed at
counterbalancing such disturbances:

πραΰνειν μὲν γὰρ προσήκει τὰ μετὰ τῶν ἀγρυπνιῶν, ἐπεγείρειν δὲ τὰ μετὰ τῆς
ἀκινησίας. εἰκότως οὖν ἀκμαζόντων αὐτῶν τοῖς μὲν ἀγρυπνιτικοῖς καὶ περικοπτικοῖς

[15] *Loc. Aff. 3.6. K.VIII*: 161, 15–16.

69

νοσήμασι τὰς διὰ μήκωνος κωδειῶν ἐπιβροχὰς προσοίσομεν ... καρῶσαι γὰρ χρὴ καὶ ναρκῶσαι ποιῆσαι το ἡγεμονικόν, ἐμψύχοντα δηλονότι τὸν ὑπερτεθερμασμένον ἐγκέφαλον. ἐπὶ δὲ τῶν ἐναντίων παθῶν ἐπεγεῖραι καὶ τέμνειν καὶ θερμῆναι προσήκει τὸ πάχος τοῦ λυποῦντος χυμοῦ ... ἐναφεψοῦντες οὖν ὄξει θύμον καὶ γλήχωνα καὶ ὀρίγανον ... τῇ ῥινὶ ... προσοίσομεν, ὅπως ὁ ἀτμὸς ἐπὶ τὸν ἐγκέφαλον ἀναφερόμενος τέμνῃ τὸ πάχος τοῦ χυμοῦ. *MM XIII.21. LCL III*: 402, 20–5; 28–8; 404, 1–3; 8–11. *K.X*: 930–1.

It is convenient to soothe those who are sleepless, and to stimulate those who are motionless. We can reasonably administer washings with poppy heads when diseases with insomnia and delirium peak ... for it is necessary to make the ruling part (*hêgemonikon*) somnolent and numb by cooling the evidently over-heated brain. In the opposite affection it is appropriate to revive, to thin and to heat the thickness of the distressed humour ... We should apply thyme, penny-royal and oregano boiled with vinegar ... to the nose ... so that the vapour carried up to the brain can thin the thick humour.

We have already seen several of these elements in Aretaeus' discussion: the thickness, the heat or coldness of the humour according to the affection, and the intervention of *atmos*. However, in his eclectic approach it was not so clear how they interacted, nor was the way in which the treatment affected the body so elaborately explained. Galen justifies carefully and specifically the mechanism of his therapies, as well as their impact on the disturbance, through his theoretical model. He even explains through it the route of administration. Drugs are to be applied to the nostrils because they can easily reach the brain – the affected part – when the patient breathes in. These explanations highlight Galen's constant interest in rationality, particularly when contrasted with Celsus' or the author of the *Anonymus Parisinus*. Even when they recommend similar products (for example, poppy), they only consider the effects, with no attention whatsoever on the kind of interaction that the drug produces.[16]

---

[16] *si nihilo minus vigilant quidam somnum moliuntur potui dando aquam, in qua papaver aut hyosciamos decocta sint* ('If they are not less wakeful [despite the previous treatments], some attempt [to achieve] sleep by giving them water to drink, in which poppy or henbane have been boiled', *Med. 3.18*: 12).
ὑπνωτικοῖς δὲ χρησόμεθα προσκλύσμασι τῷ διὰ κωδυῶν ἢ ὑοσκυάμου ἀφεψήματι ('We shall use hypnotic lotions with decoction of poppy seeds or henbane', *Anon. Paris. I.3, 7*: 6, 25–6). Aretaeus' explanation of poppy is not much more clarifying: ἐπὶ μᾶλλον δὲ ὑπνωτικὸν μήκων ἀφεψηθεῖσα ἐν λίπαϊ ἔς τε τὸ τῆς κεφαλῆς βρέγμα ('Particularly hypnotic is [applying] poppy boiled in fat to the front part of the head', *CA I.1. CMG (H).V*: 94, 19–20).

Galen's use of opium as an analgesic is also useful in contrasting his understanding of drowsiness and anaesthesia as separate – even if often simultaneous – phenomena. Unlike Celsus, who considered them both as one and the same thing (therefore he considered that *papaver* cured pain through sleep),[17] Galen distinguishes different mechanisms through which opium produces sleep and relieves pain that is resistant to treatment.

εἰ δὲ καὶ τοῦτο ἀδύνατον, διὰ τῆς τῶν ναρκωτικῶν φαρμάκων προσφορᾶς ... λεπτὰ γὰρ ὑπάρχει ταῖς συστάσεσι καὶ θερμὰ ταῖς δυνάμεσι τὰ πλεῖστα τῶν τοιούτων ὑγρῶν· ὅσα δὲ δι' ὀπίου καὶ ὑοσκυάμου ... σκευάζεται φάρμακα, ψύχει τε ἅμα καὶ ξηραίνει πάντως ... οὐ μόνον ὡς αἰσθήσεως ναρκωτικὰ χρήσιμα καθέστηκεν, ἀλλὰ καὶ ὡς συνιστάντα καὶ παχύνοντα τὴν τῶν ὑγρῶν λεπτότητα καὶ προσέτι καὶ τὴν θερμότητα σφοδρὰν ὑπάρχουσαν ἐμψύχοντα. *MM XII.8. LCL III*: 300, 8–13. *K*: 862.

If this [therapeutic measure] is also impossible, the administration of some narcotic drug [is required] ... The majority of such humours [the humours of patients with pain that is resistant to treatment] are thin in consistency and hot in capacity. The remedies that are prepared with poppy-juice and henbane, simultaneously and fully cool and dry ... Not only do they produce a useful numbing of perception, but they also cause the combination and thickening of the thin humours. Additionally, they cool the excessive heat that predominates.

While in the discussion on delirium the drug seems to be useful because it cools the overheated brain, the relief of pain needs, apart from its cooling capacity, its drying and thickening powers too. Once again humoural physiology is at the centre of the explanation both of the disease and its treatment.

The basics of this theory are outlined in *On the causes of diseases*, where Galen establishes the correspondence between the humours and their qualities.[18] In *On the difference of diseases* Galen explains that the imbalance (*duskrasia*) of such qualities is the necessary cause of an illness.[19] However, in his personal

---

[17] This matter will be further discussed in the analysis of sleep.

[18] ἡ μὲν ξανθὴ χολὴ θερμὴ καὶ ξηρὰ τὴν δύναμίν ἐστιν, ἡ δὲ μέλαινα ξηρὰ καὶ ψυχρά· ὑγρὸν δὲ καὶ θερμὸν τὸ αἷμα· καὶ ψυχρὸν καὶ ὑγρὸν τὸ φλέγμα ('The yellow bile is hot and dry in capacity, whereas the black [bile], dry and cold. Moist and hot is blood, and cold and moist is phlegm', *Caus. Morb. 6. K.VII*: 21, 16–18; 22, 1).

[19] εἰ δ' ἐν εὐκρασίᾳ θερμοῦ καὶ ψυχροῦ καὶ ξηροῦ καὶ ὑγροῦ τὸ ὑγιαίνειν ἐστίν, ἐν τῇ τούτων δυσκρασίᾳ καὶ τὸ νοσεῖν ἐξ ἀνάγκης συμβήσεται ('If health is balance (*eukrasia*) of heat and cold, and dry and moisture, by necessity, disease will be accompanied by imbalance (*duskrasia*) of these', *Morb. Diff. 2. K.VI*: 838, 12–15).

reading of Hippocrates neither all humours, nor all qualities have the same status.[20] There seems to be a hierarchy:

... ἔγκαυσίς τε καὶ ψύξις τῆς κεφαλῆς ἐνδείκνυται ταὐτόν· ἀγρυπνητικαὶ μὲν αἱ ἐγκαύσεις, καταφορικαὶ δ' αἱ ψύξεις γινόμεναι. καὶ μὴν καὶ τὰ χολώδη τῶν νοσημάτων καὶ θερμὰ τὰς ἀγρυπνίας καὶ παραφροσύνας καὶ φρενίτιδας ἐργαζόμενα φαίνεται· τούτοις δ' ἔμπαλιν τὰ φλεγματικὰ καὶ ψυχρὰ νωθρότητάς τε καὶ καταφοράς. ἡ μὲν πρώτη δύναμις ἐν τῇ κατὰ τὸ θερμόν τε καὶ ψυχρόν ἐστι δυσκρσίᾳ, τῶν ἀγρυπνητικῶν τε καὶ καταφορικῶν νοσημάτων· ἐφεξῆς δ' αὐτῆς ἡ καθ' ὑγρότητα καὶ ξηρότητα. τά τε γὰρ λουτρὰ πάντας ὑπνώδεις ἐργάζεται τὴν κεφαλὴν ὑγραίνοντα, καὶ οἴνου πόσις εὔκρατος, καὶ ὑγραίνουσαι τροφαὶ πᾶσαι ... ταῦτ' οὖν ἅπαντα τεκμήρια γενέσθω τοῦ δευτέραν μὲν ἔχειν χώραν εἰς ἀργίαν ψυχῆς τὴν παρὰ φύσιν ὑγρότητα, προτέραν δ' αὐτῆς εἶναι τὴν ψυχρότητα. *Loc. Aff. 3, 6. K.VIII*: 161, 14–19; 162, 1–6, 8–10.

... The heating up and cooling down of the head can demonstrate this: heat triggers insomnia, whereas coldness triggers drowsiness (*kataphora*). Also, the bilious and hot diseases seem to produce insomnia, delirium (*paraphrosunas*) and *phrenitis*, as opposed to phlegmatic and cold [ones, which cause] sluggish (*nôthrotêtas*) and drowsy (*kataphoras*) conditions. The main [affected] capacity of sleepless and drowsy diseases resides in the imbalance (*duskrasia*) of heat and cold, subsequently in that [in the *duskrasia*] of moist and dry. Indeed, baths are sleep-inducing for everybody, for they moisten the head, as is drinking well-tempered wine, and all the wet nourishment ... Let all this be a proof that moistness opposite to nature has the second position in causing idleness of the *psuchê*, whilst coldness has the first.

For certain, bile and phlegm are more frequently mentioned in these kinds of diseases, and the pair hot–cold seems to have pre-eminence over dry–moist. Moreover, the antithetic character of the humours and their qualities enables Galen to explain with a persuasive logic the opposite nature of certain symptoms, such as insomnia–drowsiness. In other words, what we nowadays consider as hyperactive impaired consciousness is associated by Galen with heat, whereas hypoactive impaired consciousness is associated with coldness. By distinguishing two hierarchies in the status of the contrasting pairs of qualities, he adds complexity to the theory, thereby increasing the level of expertise required to treat the conditions.

---

[20] Even though *On the nature of man* – where the theory of the four humours is most clearly expounded upon – is nowadays attributed to Polybus, Hippocrates' son-in-law, Galen believed it to be genuinely Hippocratic (Nutton 2008: 147).

The humoural theory is further complicated by Galen's gradual understanding of it. In this sense, I disagree with Jouanna's hypothesis of the dual nature of madness that he finds to be similar to the Hippocratic corpus.[21] On the contrary, Galen conceives the qualities of humours as a continuum where properties are dependent on the gradation of a certain quality:

ὅτ' ἄν δ' ἐν αὐτῷ πλεονάσῃ τῷ του ἐγκεφάλου σώματι, μελαγχολίαν ἐργάζεται, καθάπερ ὁ ἕτερος χυμὸς τῆς μελαίνης χολῆς, ὁ κατωπτημένης τῆς ξανθῆς χολῆς γενόμενος, τὰς θηριώδεις παραφροσύνας ἀποτελεῖ χωρὶς πυρετοῦ τε καὶ συν πυρετῷ, πλεονάζων ἐν τῷ σώματι τοῦ ἐγκεφάλου. καὶ διὰ τοῦτο τῆς φρενίτιδος ἡ μὲν τίς ἐστι μετριωτέρα, τὴν γένεσιν ἐκ τῆς ὠχρᾶς ἔχουσα χολῆς· ἡ δέ τις σφοδροτέρα, τῆς ξανθῆς ἔγγονος ὑπάρχουσα· καί τις ἄλλη θηριώδης τε καὶ μελαγχολικὴ παραφροσύνη γίνεται κατοπτηθείσης τῆς ξανθῆς χολῆς. *Loc. Aff.* *3.9. K.VIII*: 177, 15–17; 178, 1–7.

Whenever [black bile] is in excess in the body of the brain, it produces *melancholy*, just like the other black bile humour that originates in the concoction of yellow bile, which – by excessive accumulation in the body of the brain – causes wild delirium (*paraphrosunas*), with or without fever. This is the reason why one type of *phrenitis* is more moderate: because its origin is pale bile; whereas a more violent type is the result of yellow [bile]. There is yet another wild and *melancholic* delirium (*thêriôdês te kai melancholikê paraphrosunê*) that is generated when the yellow bile is concocted.

In this way, humours have simultaneously a qualitative and quantitative dimension that determines the specific characteristics of diseases. The degree of their violence is, in this case, directly related to the darkness of the bile.[22] Accordingly, the treatment should compensate for the degree of distortion. In Galen's own words: δύο εἰσὶν οὗτοι σκοποὶ περί τε τὸ ὑγιεινὸν καὶ τὸ νοσερόν, ἡ ποιότης τε καὶ ἡ ποσότης τοῦ προσφερομένου ('there are two aims

---

[21] Jouanna (2013: 113) fails to see that Galen had a gradual rather than binary view of what he defines as 'madness' (which we have defined as impaired consciousness). The following passage supports the idea that a progression in the qualities of the humours is considered to cause a proportional increase in the severity of the symptoms.

[22] Of note are the Hippocratic echoes of this passage. I have mentioned before the usefulness of bathing the head in delirious *phrenitic* patients (*Aff. LCL 10*), which had a long tradition, for Celsus, Aretaeus and the *Anonymus Parisinus* also recommend it. This is also the case in this passage, where the different shades of bile determine the severity of the ailment (which reminds us of *Morb. I. LCL 30*: 158, 5–6; 9–11; 13–16). Devinant (2020: 225–6) offers an interesting review of the physiology and effects of the different types of bile.

concerning health and disease: the quality and the quantity of what needs to be provided').[23] Further down he expands:

... ἐὰν δέκα μὲν ἀριθμοῖς ἐπὶ τὸ θερμότερον ἐξεστήκῃ τοῦ κατὰ φύσιν, ἑπτὰ δ' ἐπὶ τὸ ξηρότερον· εἶναι δήπου χρὴ καὶ τὸ ὑγιεινὸν αἴτιον ἐπὶ ταῖς τοιαύταις διαθέσεσι δέκα μὲν ἀριθμοῖς ψυχρότερον, ἑπτὰ δὲ ὑγρότερον· *Ars. Med. CUF 28.15*: 363, 17; 364, 1–4. *K*: 383.

... If [the *duskrasia*] has deviated from the norm by ten numbers towards the hotter, and by seven towards the drier, it would – of course – be necessary, for the cause that brings about health in such conditions to be ten times colder, and seven times moister.

The actual interaction of all these ideas can be clearly seen in Galen's self-promoting anecdote regarding his discovery of the treatment for memory loss:

ἐκ τίνος, Ἀρχίγενες, λόγου πιθανοῦ πεισθέντες ἐπὶ τὴν κεφαλὴν ἀφιξόμεθα τὴν καρδίαν ἀφέντες, ἧς ἕν μὲν τι τῶν συμφύτων ἔργων ἐστὶν τὸ μεμνῆσθαι, τὸ πάθος δὲ τῆς ἐνεργείας ἐστὶν ἡ ταύτης ἀπώλεια; τίνα δὲ διάθεσιν ἡ τῇ κεφαλῇ προσφερομένη σικύα θεραπεύουσα τὴν μνήμην ἀνακελέσεται;...

τὸ δὲ σικύαις μόναις κεχρῆσθαι χάριν μὲν τοῦ θερμῆναι χρήσιμον, ἄλλως δ' οὐδαμῶς· ἐπισπῶνται γὰρ ἐκ τοῦ βάθους εἰς αὐτὰ αἱ σικύαι τὴν ὑγρότητα ...

ὡς εἶναι δῆλον αὐτὸν ὑγρότητα καὶ ψύξιν ἡγούμενον εἶναι τὴν διάθεσιν ἤτοι κατὰ τὸν ἐγκέφαλον, ἢ τὰς μήνιγγας· οὐ γὰρ δὴ κατά γε τὸ κρανίον ἡ τοιαύτη διάθεσις γενομένη τῆς μνήμης ἀφαιρήσεται τὸν ἄνθρωπον. *Loc. Aff. 3.5. K.VIII*: 151, 4–9; 152, 3–5; 153, 14–18.

Based on which persuasive reasoning, Archigenes, are you going to convince us to get hold of the head and disregard the heart, one of whose innate actions is to remember, and whose activity is destroyed when affected?[24] By curing which condition will the cupping-glass applied to the head bring back the memory?...

The use of the cupping-glass on its own is useful in order to heat, but nothing else. The cupping-glass sucks up the humidity from the depths towards itself...

It is evident that he [Archigenes] believed that a humid and cold condition was affecting the brain and the meninges, for such a condition in the skull could not deprive a person of his memory.

---

[23] *Ars. Med. CUF 23.13*: 348, 16, 7; 349, 1. *K.I*: 369.
[24] As evidenced by this *reductio ad absurdum*, Archigenes of Apamea was probably a supporter of cardiocentric theories (at least that is what Galen is implying), which makes sense considering that he was a disciple of Athenaeus of Attaleia (Nutton 2013a: 203). It should be emphasised that Galen is not so much questioning the recommended treatment as he is mocking the incorrect rationale for such treatment.

This criticism of Archigenes is another case where anatomy indicates the site to apply the treatment (the specific location in the brain and meninges as opposed to the skull probably suggests a stronger remedy, for it needs to reach deeper). More importantly, though, the nature of the quality imbalance is crucial for deciding the kind of treatment. The cupping-glass, with its heating and drying effects, can only be justified for cold and moist conditions, in a clear example of opposites cure opposites.

Once again, Galen's impressive achievement was articulating into a coherent whole the allegedly Hippocratic views concerning humours and qualities, with some Platonic and Aristotelian theorisations about the four elements, and with the latest discoveries of the Alexandrian anatomical revival.[25] In this way, he found a logical rationale for several treatments that were widely accepted because of their long historical tradition, and used this advantage to criticise his competitors, who could offer no coherent explanation, even if they chose those same therapies. In other words, this solid system, which conceived a tight and self-contained notion of illness, enabled Galen to build authority in the highly competitive and cultivated milieu that he inhabited.

---

[25] As other authors have also argued: Schöner (1964: 65), Smith (1979: 63–5, 124), Hankinson (2008: 11).

CHAPTER 6

FINAL REMARKS ABOUT DELIRIUM AND THE NOTION OF DISEASE: A DIACHRONIC LOOK

This analysis has challenged a rather unanimous assumption of current scholarship, which frames ancient descriptions of delirium as mental illness.[1] It proposes instead to delimit a specific clinical presentation – hyperactive impaired consciousness – as an alternative category that better describes – with fewer anachronistic theoretical assumptions – most of the cases that scholars have so far perceived as madness. This finding might seem particularly controversial when applied to the Hippocratic corpus, for contrary to an important scholarly tradition,[2] I propose that the vast majority of descriptions are addressing cases of delirium, whereas madness was rarely discussed. Similarly, from the post-Hellenistic sources onwards, although I agree with most scholars that medical texts did discuss madness,[3] I consider mental illness and wakeful impaired consciousness as two different types of entities that needed to be distinguished.

In light of these findings, the tendency in contemporary scholarship to force a modern construct such as mental illness onto ancient narratives seems to be rather misleading. Indeed, although it is possible to find some coincidences and draw certain parallels, our conception of mental illness is so deeply theory-laden that it can hardly be extrapolated to the ancient medical texts. As a result, when researchers assume the validity of these categories they end up grouping and classifying the ancient material in ways that do not necessarily reflect their original conceptions. Impaired consciousness, conversely, which is clinically closer to our definition of a syndrome rather than to a fully fledged disease, is easier to recognise and presupposes fewer theoretical assumptions.

---

[1] Particularly, Pigeaud (1987) and most of the articles in Harris' (2013) volume start from this premise without actually debating it. Many other scholars also make similar assumptions: van der Eijk (2005), Matentzoglu (2011), Thumiger (2013).

[2] di Benedetto (1986), Matentzoglu (2011), Jouanna (2013), Thumiger (2017).

[3] Pigeaud (1994), Stok (1996), Murphy (2013), Nutton (2013b), McDonald (2014).

In this sense, the clear distinction between impaired consciousness and madness presents us with new challenges. Considering the strong emphasis put by the authors (particularly the post-Hellenistic ones) on the differential diagnosis between these two conditions, questions should be raised concerning the relevance of such a distinction. Beyond the evident impact that it had in terms of therapy within medical discourse, contrasting delirium with madness might also have been important in other disciplines.[4]

In terms of chronological changes, our analysis of wakeful impaired consciousness in general and *phrenitis* in particular shows how they were conceived, how their understanding evolved in the studied sources and how the notion of disease mutated in parallel with those changes. Overall, we can see a persistent tension between theory and clinic, and a progressive trend away from concrete symptomatic descriptions towards more abstract conceptualisations.

In the Hippocratic corpus the tension leaned towards the clinical end. Most descriptions of impaired consciousness show a certain laxity in the notion of illness, by giving pre-eminence to thorough and detailed clinical accounts over more abstract association of symptoms with distinct diseases. This is particularly evident in the books of *Epidemics*, where most cases are comprised of catastases and detailed descriptions (most of them without a specific name). But even in the nosological treatises – where allegedly individual diseases such as *phrenitis* (and also *lethargy*) are tackled – the boundaries between the different conditions tend to be less emphasised than in later works. Hippocratic authors grouped *phrenitis* with other related diseases that required a similar kind of care[5] (particularly with *peripneumonia* and *pleuritis*).[6] In this way, the notion of disease that emerges from these authors is loose, non-specific, and it mostly consists of collections of manifestations rather than abstract nosological entities.[7]

---

[4] I have elsewhere discussed how legal notions such as responsibility, competence and capacity were very much dependent on understanding the difference between these two types of affection (Pelavski, 2023: 399–426). It could be interesting, perhaps, to explore the implications of this distinction in other areas of knowledge and culture.

[5] With acute ones (*Acut. CUF*: 5), or with diseases of the cavity (*Aff. LCL*: 6).

[6] *Morb. III. LCL*: 15, and *Aff. LCL*: 10.

[7] To use Pigeaud's terms, 'subsuming the symptoms into a concept is not essential for the Hippocratic doctor' (1981: 257).

In post-Hellenistic treatises this emphasis slightly shifts towards theory; we could claim that there was a growing focalisation on certain symptoms, paralleled by a progressive development towards their conceptual abstraction. Of the large Hippocratic list of symptoms, some gained increasing attention, whereas there is growing indifference towards several others. Such is the case of speech disorders and coma vigil, which paled into insignificance (especially in Aretaeus' work, where the latter is not even described, while in Celsus it appears only once).[8] On the contrary, the relevance of insomnia grew remarkably in close association with the presentation of *phrenitis*,[9] and so did hallucinations.

As discussed, impaired consciousness in *On medicine* was directly related to the *vanas imagines* (hallucinations); however, they were construed as a crucial symptom rather than its main cause. In Aretaeus, perception *(aisthêsis)* becomes a totally independent principle,[10] and it is its impairment (manifested through hallucinations) that triggers diseases with a compromised consciousness. In

---

[8] *sin cerebrum membranave eius vulnus accepit ... quorundam sensus optunduntur, appellatique ignorant; quorundam trux vultus est; quorundam oculi quasi resoluti huc atque illuc moventur; fereque tertio vel quinto die delirium accedit* ('If the brain or its membrane gets injured ... their sensations become powerless: they do not respond when they are called; in others, the expression of their faces becomes threatening; and yet in others the eyes move here and there as though they were without restraint. Often during the third or fifth day, delirium appears', *Med. 5.26*: 14). Although strictly speaking the author is separating vigil coma from delirium as two different stages within the same disease, they are discussed as related phenomena.

[9] *Lethargy* underwent the same process but with the opposite sign. In the HC it is construed as an acute winter disease – like *pneumonia* or *pleurisy* (*Aph. LCL III.23*: 130) – where stupor *(kôma)* is one amid many other symptoms including cough, moist sputum, weakness and liquid stools before death (*Morb. III. LCL 5*: 12, 5–10). This clinical description is confirmed by the authors of *Coan Prenotions* (*Coac. LCL 136*: 134, 6–8) and *Diseases II*, who also adds that the patient 'talks nonsense, and when he finishes talking nonsense he falls asleep' (*Morb. II. CUF 65*: 267, 14). In other words, among the Hippocratic doctors *lethargy* presents some form of drowsiness but not as its key sign. On the other hand, just as *phrenitis* started to be consistently defined by insomnia and wakefulness in post-Hellenistic treatises, so did *lethargy* with sleepiness and drowsy impaired consciousness. Particularly explicit about this is the *Anonymus Parisinus*, where some Hippocratic ideas were expanded, thereby turning drowsy impaired consciousness into the main symptom of the disease: 'they do not reply easily ... they are delirious ... involuntary urine and stools' (*Anon. Paris. II.2, 2*: 12, 5–7; *II.2, 5*: 12, 12). The tendency persisted throughout the later tradition, including *Medical definitions* (*Def. Med. 235. K.XIX*: 413, 5–9), *Introduction* (*Introd. CUF XIII.25*: 51, 22–4) and – as already discussed – in Celsus (*Med. 3.20*: 1), Aretaeus (*CA I.2. CMG (H).V*: 98, 8–14) and Galen (*Hipp. Com. 3,1. K.VII*: 656).

[10] The issue is further discussed in the section on HOFs in Part II.

other words, the growth in relevance of this symptom within the medical discourse is accompanied by a progressively abstract reflection on perceptions.[11]

This process of privileging certain features to the detriment of certain others also reveals the way in which illnesses became better defined notions with stricter boundaries. As Pigeaud has remarked, post-Hellenistic works placed a strong focus on nosological taxonomy. In this way, contrary to the Hippocratic corpus, these treatises put their emphasis on diseases, which were organised into comprehensive classificatory systems based on a restricted number of symptoms.[12] Undoubtedly, this novel theoretical framework required adapting the vague and broad notion of impaired consciousness into smaller categories, and encouraged doctors to funnel the complexities of delirium into stricter classifications that often used opposing symptoms as dichotomous sorting criteria:[13] acute versus chronic, with or without fever, wakeful versus somnolent, affecting the head or the heart, etc. This tendency to compartmentalise diseases is present – to a greater or lesser extent – in all the post-Hellenistic authors discussed, and the challenge for these doctors was to adapt the vast Hippocratic clinical diversity to the available classifications and possible explanations, where symptoms, affected organs, physio-pathological mechanisms and treatments were more cohesively grouped. In this sense, Celsus' encyclopaedism and Aretaeus' lax eclecticism are different approaches with the same aim.

Galen will take matters further. In his systematisation of the *psuchê*, perceptions are also an independent activity (or HOF to use our contemporary terminology), but they are not the primary problem. They are vicariously compromised by an affection of the ruling part, a concept with an even higher level of abstraction: it is in the *hêgemonikon* that the problem actually occurs. Furthermore, the symptom-focused definition of disease turned

---

[11] Possibly, this shift of emphasis was related to the Hellenistic advances in the understanding of the nervous system, and mirrored the ongoing philosophical debates on *aisthêsis* and its relation to reality. Considerations of such issues were well within the intellectual zeitgeist, as Pigeaud (1987: 95–9) has thoroughly analysed in his discussion on *phantasia, phantaston, phantasticon* and *phantasma*.

[12] Pigeaud (1987: 81).

[13] I have argued that Aretaeus' lax eclecticism enabled him to be less conditioned by these constraints as compared to the other post-Hellenistic authors (although not completely free).

Final remarks about delirium and the notion of disease

into an activity-focused one. This author conceived illnesses as the impairment of certain activities (*energeiai*), which in turn depended on the conditions of the body (*diatheseis*) that enabled such activities.

συγχωρείτωσαν ἡμῖν . . . οὐχ ἅπασαν τὴν παρὰ φύσιν διάθεσιν, ἀλλ᾽ ἥτις ἂν ἐνέργειαν βλάπτῃ νόσημα προσαγορεύειν· ἥτις δ᾽ ἂν παρὰ φύσιν μὲν ᾖ, μὴ μέντοι βλάπτῃ γ᾽ ἐνέργειαν, οὐ νόσον, ἀλλὰ σύμπτωμα νοσήματος. *MM I.9. LCL I:* 110, 27–8; 112, 1–3. *K.X:* 71.

I should be allowed to . . . designate as 'disease' not every condition contrary to nature but those where an activity is damaged. When, conversely, there are conditions contrary to nature but they do not damage an activity, they are not an illness but its symptom.

The relevance of concrete symptoms as the key elements to define and classify diseases has waned and been replaced by a more abstract concept, namely, the activity. Unlike the post-Hellenistic therapeutic approach, Galen's method did not target the symptoms but the abnormal *diathesis* that was hindering a specific *energeia*. Accordingly, τό γέ τοι τῆς θεραπείας δεόμενον οὐδὲν ἄλλο ἐστὶ πλὴν τῆς βλαπτούσης τὴν ἐνέργειαν διαθέσεως ('nothing else but the condition (*diathesis*) that damages the activity (*energeia*) needs treatment').[14] Thus, diseases were conceptually reframed. The complexities of the diagnosis of *phrenitis* still required there to be fever and delirium (among other symptoms).[15] However, for Galen that implied a combination of θερμότης ὡς ἤδη βλάπτειν ἐνέργειαν ('heat that was such as to damage an activity (*energeia*)')[16] – i.e. Galen´s definition of fever – accompanied by πλημμελεῖς . . . κινήσεις τῆς ἡγεμονικῆς δυνάμεως, ἐπὶ μοχθηροῖς συνίστανται χυμοῖς ἢ δυσκρασίᾳ τῶν κατὰ τὸν ἐγκέφαλον ('a defective movement of the *hegemonic* capacities secondary to pernicious humours or *duskrasia* in the brain')[17] – that is, Galen's definition of delirium. Thus, the symptoms were only relevant as long as they provided information about the *diathesis* of the body that was impairing the *energeia*, whereas the name of the diseases was merely

---

[14] *MM I.9. LCL:* 108, 1–2. *K.X:* 69.
[15] κείσθω τοίνυν κατ᾽ ἀμφοῖν τούτοιν ἓν ὄνομα, τὸ πυρέττειν λέγω καὶ παραφρονεῖν, καὶ καλείσθω φρενιτικὸς ὁ τοιοῦτος ('I say: let one name be attributed to both, the feverish and delirious person, and let that person be called *phrenitic*', *MM II.7. LCL I:* 230, 24–6. *K.X:* 149).
[16] *MM II.7. LCL I. K.X:* 150, 22.   [17] *Caus. Symp. II, 7. K.VII:* 202, 3–5.

a simplified way to group relevant symptoms. Conveniently, both the excessive heat and the abnormal humours could be targeted by Galenic medicine.

As a matter of fact, up until Galen, treatments were conceived as lists of actions or drugs (getting married, purgation, beatings, changes in illumination, etc.) aimed at palliating symptoms and mainly based on previous experience or common sense. Depending on the notion of disease, such catalogues of instructions were more or less specific for a kind of condition. Only seldom (occasionally with Aretaeus) can one see a physio-pathological rationale behind a specific therapy. It is with Galen that combating the cause becomes the main (and often the only) objective of the treatment, which was strictly informed by his tripartite understanding of disease, where the *locus affectus* dictated the site of application, and the type and magnitude of the *duskrasia* indicated the kind and potency of the remedies.[18]

In other words, Galen – despite his thorough symptomatic accounts – took the tension between theory and clinic to the more abstract end. The Hippocratic writers' detailed clinical descriptions, and the post-Hellenistic attempts to delimit distinct nosological entities shared a common interest in the patient and their clinical presentations, even if they put a different emphasis on each component. Galen's approach, on the other hand, regarded the individual as a collection of organs and humours aimed at fulfilling certain activities (*energeiai*), and most of his attention was focused on finding correlations between impaired activities and alterations in these components.[19] In his coherent and cohesive theoretical system, diseases presented symptoms emerging from altered functions in specific bodily parts, which could be explained by mechanisms (mostly humoural), the correction of which required corresponding treatments. (It is in this sense that the focus is placed on theory, and

---

[18] In this sense I disagree with McDonald (2009a: 147) that Galen's 'theory of treatment is very complex', or that he seems 'to neglect humoural theory altogether' (153).

[19] Although I do not disagree with Devinant's five Galenic criteria for defining 'psychic diseases' (Devinant, 2020: 102–5), highlighting the three pillars of his system (*locus affectus*, type of *duskrasia* and degree of alteration of qualities) makes it simpler to understand his rationale for most of his treatments, and his choice to distinguish certain conditions and not others.

the clinical presentations are only relevant as long as they can reveal the more abstract mechanisms underlying the problem.)

In contrast to the changes in the notion of disease that emerge from the analysis of wakeful impaired consciousness throughout the different periods, there are also features that remained stable. We could argue that what we nowadays designate as delirium could be identified – to a greater or lesser degree – by all the ancient sources under analysis as a variable and intermittent state of abnormal behaviour, often accompanied by altered perceptions, which could sometimes be triggered by wine (and other substances), fever or certain acute conditions. Although it could appear in the midst of longer infirmities (such as diseases of young virgins in the HC or *melancholia* from the post-Hellenistic sources onwards), it was construed as a recognisable entity that often needed to be distinguished from conditions nowadays identified as mental illness.

PART II

SLEEP

.

CHAPTER 7

A GENERAL GLANCE AT SLEEP

After looking at delirium – mostly from the hyperactive end of the spectrum of consciousness – in this part I shall explore the hypoactive end, particularly sleep. This second ideal exemplar, which is a universal process, intrinsic to human existence, also presents challenges in terms of boundaries. Just as the fuzzy edges between delirium and mental illness enabled us to reflect upon the chronological changes in the notion of disease, the analysis of sleep will help us deepen our inquiry into the blurry boundaries between health and illness. Additionally, questioning the terminology used to describe alterations at both ends of the spectrum of consciousness and their recovery will be useful in understanding some of these doctors' ideas about the mind.

Sleep has often been construed as a vaguely defined territory with fuzzy edges, in the midst of apparently contradictory tensions: beyond the difficulty in establishing when it should be regarded as a normal physiological process and when as a sign of disease, the boundaries that separate it from drowsiness and hypoactive wakeful impaired consciousness, on the one hand, and from total loss of consciousness, on the other, are rather blurry.[1] In other words, even the apparently self-evident contrast between wakefulness and sleep can be tricky. To quote Williams, sleep 'furnishes us with a sense of what it means to be conscious, just as consciousness furnishes us with a sense of what it means to be asleep'.[2]

To address these ambiguities – not always resolved by the medical texts – apart from the biological approach I will consider in my analysis some recent contributions by other disciplines, which have also explored the phenomenon and engaged in similar debates. Sleep is becoming an increasingly important field of research

---

[1] Even nowadays these tensions are not devoid of dilemmas (Thorarinsdottir et al., 2019).
[2] Williams (2008: 640–1).

among sociologists and anthropologists, whose perspectives often illuminate relevant areas that medicine leaves in the dark.

In a pioneering paper, Taylor proposed to study sleep as a social rather than a biological phenomenon. He suggested that only physiology and medicine had addressed the topic so far, and their questions were only aimed at the 'whats' and 'whys'. He claimed, instead, that there were still important inquiries to be made concerning its sociological dimensions, such as 'How? When? Where? With whom? and What meanings can be attributed to sleeping?'[3] Considering that scientific ideas are often entangled with sociological beliefs, and medical concepts can be influenced by extra-medical realities, asking such questions about ancient societies can provide us with important information.

Not far from these approaches, Oberhelman offered a more anthropological take to the matter. He highlighted how sleeping, due to its inseparable link with dreaming, pervades various discourses on disease and healing in antiquity. Not only was it conceived as a symptom of disease, as part of a healthy regimen and as the treatment for certain illnesses, it also appears as a component of rituals under the form of incubation in temples, and is even associated with death in epic poems.[4]

In other words, in order to explore the different ancient medical writers' perceptions of sleep and their link to reduced/impaired consciousness – or unconsciousness – my analysis will place the phenomenon against a background of sociological and anthropological realities.[5] Such backgrounds will both inform the medical discourse and help us to define the fuzzy contours of sleep. Undoubtedly, the tensions wakefulness–sleep and health–disease confer a liminal status to this clinical presentation.[6] Furthermore,

---

[3] Taylor (1993: 463–71).

[4] Oberhelman (2016: 2, 6). Thumiger (2017: 177) also reminds us of the association among the ancients between sleep and death – a reversible death.

[5] The recent surge of interest in anthropological and sociological aspects of sleep has also triggered interesting contributions among classicists. See Brunt and Steger (2003), and particularly Nissin (2016), who wrote a monographic study of sleeping spaces in the Roman house.

[6] It should be noted that the ambivalence of sleep and its contradictory roles were not exclusive of the scientific discourse, but penetrated several others. As Jouanna (1983: 49–62) has convincingly argued, this counterpoint had a strong correlation in Attic drama, and the 'protective' versus 'destructive' powers of sleep were present in several tragedies.

they illuminate the peripheries of sleep; namely, the areas where the discourse on sleep intersects with other forms of impaired consciousness, thereby illuminating the extent to which authors understood them to be related or easily confusable conditions.

Additionally, this prototypical presentation enables us to explore how the authors construed different depths of sleep. As described in Chapter I, the cognitive model of classification based on ideal exemplars (chosen to define impaired consciousness) allows membership gradience. When applying this idea to sleep, one could argue that the degree of identification of any description with this prototype is inversely proportional to the level of consciousness that the author is trying to convey: the deeper a person sleeps (that is, the closer to the ideal archetype of sleep), the lower his level of consciousness. Conversely, as sleep wanes into drowsiness, the features become increasingly distant from that ideal exemplar, and accordingly, the level of consciousness increases.

Finally, this clinical presentation can also illustrate – when focusing on the terminology utilised to describe its hyper- and hypoactive peripheries – the idea of mind underlying the accounts of sleep and delirium. Accordingly, the analysis will show how the different sources perceived, described and organised the HOFs that were damaged during episodes of impaired consciousness, and how they subsumed some or many of these mental capacities within notions akin to our idea of consciousness, thereby suggesting that they had an embryonic or rudimentary intuition of this concept.

CHAPTER 8

SLEEP IN THE HIPPOCRATIC CORPUS

It seems as though scholars have paid much more attention to dreams than to sleep itself, even though allusions to the latter permeate the whole Hippocratic corpus.[1] Moreover, despite the fact that such allusions often describe patients disconnected from their surroundings, the link between sleep and impaired consciousness has been persistently overlooked.[2] In fact, the way in which this disconnection was interpreted defined how these doctors actually approached this process. Not only did it guide their stance in the debate about limits (that is, where sleep starts and wakefulness ends), but it also determined their view concerning the more theoretical challenges (namely, where each author set the boundaries between health/normality, disease/abnormality). Furthermore, as Thumiger points out, sensory perceptions allow the interaction of the body with the outside world, and the health of the mind is strongly dependent on that interaction.[3] Consequently, the disruption that occurs during sleep can also tell us about these doctors' ideas about the mind.

Disconnection and the fuzzy edges of sleep

The ambiguities in the relationship between sleep and health are ubiquitous.[4] Some authors considered sleep as a natural healthy and physiological process, others as a pathological state where

---

[1] Recent examples are Harris (2009: 174–84) and Hulskamp (2013: 33–54).

[2] Thumiger (2017: 174–88) does devote a whole chapter to sleep; however, given her broad definition of mental illness, the role of sleep in consciousness is only tangentially touched upon. Marelli's paper (1983: 331, 337), on the other hand, offers some insight into the matter, although he specifically explored how sleep is related across the corpus to the pre-Socratic philosophers, on the one hand, and to Aristotle, on the other.

[3] Thumiger (2017: 334).

[4] Byl (1998: 34) offers several examples that illustrate the ambivalence of sleep in terms of health and disease. I will focus on those where this ambivalence concerns alterations of consciousness.

consciousness was altered. There is yet a third group that distinguished between a healthy and a pathological kind of sleep. Similarly, the fuzzy edges of the notion of consciousness manifest through the fact that in certain texts there is such an overlap between hallucinations, nightmares and visions that it is difficult to know whether the writer is talking about dreams, wakeful hallucinations or intermediate states.[5]

Sleep as health

This approach is illustrated in the theoretical work *On regimen*. In book 4 sleep is described as the perfect and most active phase of the *psuchê*, where – while disconnected from the environment – κινεομένη καὶ ἐγρηγορέουσα διοικεῖ τὸν ἑωυτῆς οἶκον ('setting itself in motion and being awake, it [the *psuchê*] administers its own household').[6] Namely, by becoming detached from the outside world the *psuchê* is able to concentrate on and organise the body. Moreover, through this inwardly directed focus, it can provide, by means of dreams, valuable information about its current condition and emotional state.[7]

In a like manner, in *Aphorisms* sleep is opposed to sick conditions, which it resolves: παραφροσύνην ὕπνος παύει ('sleep puts an end to delirium').[8] Also in *Prognostic* τὴν μὲν ἡμέρην ἐγρηγορέναι χρή, τὴν δὲ νύκτα καθεύδειν·... κάκιστον δὲ μὴ κοιμᾶσθαι, μήτε τῆς νυκτὸς μήτε τῆς ἡμέρης... ὑπὸ ὀδύνης τε καὶ πόνου ἀγρυπνοίη ἂν ἢ παραφρονήσει ἀπὸ τουτέου τοῦ σημείου ('it is necessary to be awake during the day and to sleep at night', and 'worst of all is not sleeping whether by night, or by day' because in such a situation 'either are pain and distress causing insomnia, or it is followed with delirium').[9] Through the 'medicalisation' of insomnia and sleep during untimely hours, this excerpt offers a glimpse into Taylor's question 'When do we sleep?' Unlike other societies where sleep can be biphasic or

---

[5] Unlike Thumiger (2017: 296) I refuse to discuss hallucinations and nightmares as the same phenomenon because, as we shall see, there are explicit attempts in certain texts to separate them, which suggests that authors were interested in distinguishing one from the other.
[6] *Vict. CMG 4.86*: 218, 8.
[7] van der Eijk (2005: 171) has related this tradition to Orphic circles and Democritus.
[8] *Aph. LCL II.2*: 109, 15.   [9] *Prog. CUF 10.1*: 26, 6–7; *X.3*: 27, 2–5.

polyphasic,[10] this medical writer seems to be privileging a nightly and monophasic pattern of sleep. Beyond the social regulation that could be read into this passage – labelling sleep as unhealthy at any time but at night could be useful in terms of social organisation and economic production – note how the two passages are a mirror image of each other: while sleep cures delirium, insomnia causes it.[11] Namely, the identification between health and sleep here is rather strong.[12]

Sleep as disease

On the other hand, the author of *On breaths* suggests an opposing view, by considering both sleep and drunkenness as states of altered *phronêsis*.

ἡγέομαι οὐδὲν ἔμπροσθεν οὐδενὶ εἶναι μᾶλλον τῶν ἐν τῷ σώματι συμβαλλόμενον ἐς φρόνησιν ἢ τὸ αἷμα. τοῦτο δ᾽ ὅταν μὲν ἐν τῷ καθεστεῶτι μένῃ, μένει καὶ ἡ φρόνησις· ἑτεροιουμένου δὲ τοῦ αἵματος μεταπίπτει καὶ ἡ φρόνησις ... πρῶτον μέν ... ὁ ὕπνος ... μαρτυρεῖ τοῖς εἰρημένοισιν· ὅταν γὰρ ἐπέλθῃ τῷ σώματι ... καὶ τὰ ὄμματα συγκλείεται, καὶ ἡ φρόνησις ἀλλοιοῦται, δόξαι τε ἕτεραί τινες ἐνδιατρίβουσιν, ἃ δὴ ἐνύπνια καλέονται. πάλιν ἐν τῇσι μέθῃσι πλέονος ἐξαίφνης γενομένου τοῦ αἵματος μεταπίπτουσιν αἱ ψυχαὶ καὶ τὰ ἐν τῇσι ψυχῇσι φρονήματα... *Flat. CHF 14.1–2*: 121, 9–16; 122, 4–6.

I believe that nothing in the body is more favourable for anyone towards *phronêsis* than the blood: whenever it remains in a stable condition, so does the *phronêsis*; as soon as the blood is altered, *phronêsis* also changes ... First of all ... sleep ... is a testimony of what has been said. Indeed, when it falls upon the body ... the eyes close, the *phronêsis* is altered, and certain other visions linger, which are called dreams. Again, during drunkenness, when the blood suddenly increases in quantity, the *psuchai* (plural) change, and so do the *phronêmata* that are in the *psuchai*...

The link between sleep and drunkenness should remind us of the two lads described above, where alcohol abuse was associated with

[10] Brunt and Steger (2003: 16–21).
[11] This idea might have influenced the association between insomnia and *phrenitis* that we have seen in post-Hellenistic texts.
[12] Interestingly, beyond the anthropological dimension, these ideas are also resonating with other extra-medical discourses. Bartos (2015: 176) has related this passage to Democritus, who associated day-sleeping with disturbance of the body, distress of the soul, idleness and lack of education, whereas Thumiger (2017: 183–4) connects it to Attic tragedy, specifically to Sophocles' *Philoctetes* and Euripides' *Heracles*.

90

wakeful impaired consciousness. This author seemingly considered that sleep shared important similarities with those conditions. From a less medical perspective, the passage may be, again, reflecting socially regulated discourses. Just as nowadays inebriation and sleepiness are regarded as at-risk corporeal states,[13] perhaps, the negative connotation of sleep according to this author (he identifies it with alcoholic intoxication) may be related to the disapproval of excessive drinking in classical Greek culture. Along the same lines, the author of *Epidemics* *V* describes Timocrates' case, in which he fell into a deep sleep or swoon after drinking heavily, and ἐδόκει τοῖσι παρεοῦσιν ... τεθνάναι ('looked like he had died to those surrounding him'),[14] thereby relating drinking with sleeping, fainting and death. Nissin has also found the negative connotation of sleep among the Romans to be related to death and to vices.[15] The usefulness of establishing socio-medical relations in this case is that they point to specific circumstances or moments during the day, in which sleep was associated with pathology. This illuminates a boundary that otherwise seems rather confusing in the purely medical discourse, and allows us to establish a provisional sociologically informed line between healthy and abnormal sleep.

Be that as it may, it is worth highlighting that regardless of their side in the debate, the authors seem to stress disconnection from the environment as a key feature of sleep. In *On regimen 4*, this disconnection is considered as a positive condition, because it allows the *psuchê* to offer valuable information – in the form of dreams – for us to interpret (*Vict. CMG 4.86*: 2, 12–13).[16] In *On breaths*, conversely, the author suggests that any *enupnion* (that is, any conscious disconnection) is pathological, causing a detachment from reality that makes sufferers 'forget about the present evils and become hopeful about a pleasant future'.[17]

---

[13] Williams (2008: 649). [14] *Epid. V. CUF V. 2.2*: 3, 2–3. [15] Nissin (2016: 53).
[16] Debru (1982: 31) points out that 'la maladie se prépare et s'annonce dans le sommeil'. Diseases are independent from sleep, but if we have the ability to discern (*krinein*) the dreams correctly (*orthôs*), we are in a better position to understand their nature.
[17] γίνονται τῶν μὲν παρεόντων κακῶν ἐπιλήσμονες, τῶν δὲ μελλόντων ἀγαθῶν εὐέλπιδες (*Flat. CHF 14.2*: 122, 6–7).

Third position: healthy and ill kinds of sleep

The author of *On the sacred disease* adopts the third way, namely, only certain dreams and nightmares are associated with pathological states:

ἔν τε τῷ ὕπνῳ οἶδα πολλοὺς οἰμώζοντας καὶ βοῶντας, τοὺς δὲ πνιγομένους, τοὺς δὲ καὶ ἀναΐσσοντας τε καὶ φεύγοντας ἔξω καὶ παραφρονέοντας μέχρι ἐπέγρωνται, ἔπειτα δὲ ὑγιέας ἐόντας καὶ φρονέοντας ὥσπερ καὶ πρότερον. *Morb. Sacr. CUF 1.3*: 3, 10–15.

I know that during sleep many groan and scream, others choke, and yet others stand up, rush outdoors and remain delirious until they wake up. They then become healthy and rational as before.

There is a clear connection in this passage between what we would nowadays designate as 'parasomnia' and delirium. Certain abnormal kinds of sleep are equated with a condition of illness – delirium (*paraphroneontas*) – from which health and reason only return with arousal. Although the author does not explicitly mention a normal kind of sleep, we can assume that those who do not belong to the many (*pollous*) who suffer this condition are unaffected by it, hence, healthy. A comparable dichotomous attitude towards sleep can be found in *Epidemics VI*. On the one hand, there is a list of τὰ ἐν τοῖσιν ὕπνοισι παροξυνόμενα ('conditions that exacerbate with sleep');[18] on the other, sleep belongs to the catalogue of ἔθος δέ, ἐξ ὧν ὑγιαίνομεν ... ὕπνοισιν ('habits from which we become healthy')[19] – in Williams' terms, the '*healthicisation*' of sleep.

Peripheries of sleep and the boundaries of consciousness

The elusive distinction between normality and abnormality, health and disease is reinforced by the blurred boundaries between wakefulness and sleep. There are ambivalent descriptions with intermediate phenomena, where it is not clear if delirium happens with the patient awake or asleep.

... παραφρονέει˙ καὶ προφαίνεσθαί οἱ δοκέει πρὸ τῶν ὀφθαλμῶν ἑρπετὰ καὶ ἄλλα πανατοδαπὰ θηρία καὶ ὁπλῖται μαχόμενοι, καὶ αὐτὸς ἐν αὐτοῖσι δοκέει μάχεσθαι˙

---

[18] *Epid. VI. LCL 8*, 5: 262.   [19] *Epid. VI. LCL 8*, 23: 270.

Disconnection and the fuzzy edges of sleep

τοιαῦτα λέγει ὡς ὁρῶν καὶ ἐπέρχεται, καὶ ἀπειλεῖ, ἢν μή τις αὐτὸν ἐᾷ ἐξιέναι . . .
τῷδε δὲ γινώσκομεν, ὅτι ἀπὸ ἐνυπνίων ἀΐσσει καὶ φοβεῖται· ὅταν ἔννοος γένηται
ἀφηγεῖται τὰ ἐνύπνια τοιαῦτα ὁρᾶν ὁποῖα καὶ τῷ σώματι ἐποίει καὶ τῇ γλώσσῃ
ἔλεγε . . . ἔστι δ᾽ ὅτε καὶ κεῖται ἄφωνος ὅλην τὴν ἡμέρην καὶ τὴν νύκτα ἀναπνέων
ἀθρόον πολὺ τὸ πνεῦμα. ὅταν δὲ παύσηται παραφρονέων, εὐθὺς ἔννοος γίνεται, καὶ
ἢν ἐρωτᾷ τις αὐτόν, ὀρθῶς ἀποκρίνεται, καὶ γινώσκει πάντα τὰ λεγόμενα. *Int. LCL*
48. LCL: 202, 7–11; 14–22.

. . . he becomes delirious (*paraphroneei*): in front of his eyes there seem to appear
animals, all other sorts of beasts and fighting soldiers. He even thinks he is
fighting amongst them, speaks as though he could see such things and attacks
and threatens if somebody does not let him out . . . In this way we can know that
he is afraid and startled by a nightmare: when he regains consciousness (*ennoos
genêtai*), he recounts what he saw in his dreams, which corresponds with what he
did with his body and said with his tongue . . . There are also times when he lies
speechless for the whole day and night taking sudden deep breaths. When
delirium stops (*pausêtai paraphroneôn*), he immediately regains consciousness
(*ennoos ginetai*) and if somebody asks him a question he answers accurately and
is able to understand all that is said.

This passage offers a good compendium of different kinds of
alterations of consciousness: the author first talks about delirium
(*paraphroneei*), and then he seamlessly moves to sleep and nightmares (*enupnion*), without mentioning a transition, as though both
were one and the same kind of phenomenon. It should be emphasised, nevertheless, that the author is grappling to separate dreams
from wakeful hallucinations. As a result, although the findings in
both are so similar that it is difficult to tell one from the other,[20]
this doctor's attempts at distinguishing them suggest that he conceived them as two different entities.

In other words, this passage is highlighting the fuzzy edges
between two ideal prototypes of impaired consciousness (sleep
and delirium), which become even more blurred when analysing
the vocabulary of recovery or 'lucidity' (to use Pigeaud's terms).[21]
The terminology used to refer to the interruption of the nightmare
(in other words, to waking up) is exactly the same as the author later
uses to mention the end of the delirium, namely, *ennoos ginomai*.

---

[20] Our model of alertness, connectedness and responsiveness explains this difficulty more
clearly, for in both states – that is, wakeful hallucinations and vivid nightmares –
alertness is present, but connectedness disturbed.

[21] Pigeaud (1987: 15).

Ultimately, both processes – nightmares and hallucinations – and their recovery seem to be framed as similar and related phenomena, because waking up and becoming *compos mentis* were expressed with the same terms.

This and the other above-mentioned cases, where sleep is associated with a terminology akin to wakeful impaired consciousness (*phronêsis allioutai, Flat. CHF 14.2*: 122, 4–6; *paraphroneontas, Morb. Sacr. CUF 1.3*: 3, 12) point towards wakeful impaired consciousness as a peripheral phenomenon of sleep, hinting that delirium should be understood as being beyond the outer edge of sleep.

There are other examples that illustrate a similar ambiguity between sleep and total loss of consciousness. In *Epidemics V*, thirty-year-old Appellaeus from Larissa had a disease that affected him at night after dinner:[22]

τῇ δὲ ἐπιούσῃ νυκτὶ ἡ νοῦσος ἐπέλαβε δεδειπνηκότα ἀπὸ πρώτου ὕπνου, καὶ εἶχε τὴν νύκτα καὶ τὴν ἡμέρην μέχρι δορπηστοῦ ἢ ἔθανε πρὶν ἐμφρονῆσαι. *Epid. V. CUF 22.4*: 14, 12–15.

The following night the disease seized him, after having dined, as soon as he went to sleep. It persisted during the night and following day until the evening. He died before coming round (*emphronêsai*).

In this passage, sleep seems to be in the peripheries of (or poorly distinguished from) total loss of consciousness. Again, the vocabulary of recovery gives testimony to that: instead of *egeirô* or *epegeirô* (the most common Hippocratic terms to convey the idea of waking up) the use of the verb *emphronêsai* suggests that the writer conceived this *hupnos* as a loss of consciousness rather than normal sleep, and therefore waking up can be equated with coming round.

So far, the examples suggest that these medical writers conceived disturbed sleep and delirium, on the one hand, and deep sleep and fainting, on the other, as related clinical signs (or as phases of similar processes) beyond the normal and physiological type of sleep. A comparable phenomenon can be found between delirium

---

[22] Many scholars have assumed that the author is describing a case of epilepsy (Lo Presti, 2013: 207, n. 43; Jouanna, 2000: 135, n. 9).

and fainting. Thynus' son in *Epidemics VII* regained consciousness (*ephronei*) after his swoon (*apsuchiê*).[23] Therefore, while sudden loss of consciousness (*apsuchiê*) was conceived as a temporary disconnection from the environment, coming round is referred to as the recovery of cognitive capacities (*phroneô*). In other words, the recuperation from fainting is expressed with the same terminology as the recovery from wakeful impaired consciousness, which again suggests that in the Hippocratic texts, delirium and swoons were different forms of 'not *phronein*' or 'not being in their (right) minds',[24] or conversely, that becoming *compos mentis* and coming round were identical processes.

To sum up, the type of disconnection that characterised agitated sleep was perceived by these Hippocratic doctors as a disorder, which they tried to distinguish from wakeful impaired consciousness and from normal healthy sleep. On the other end of the spectrum, the disconnection that occurred during deep dreamless sleep could be easily confused with fainting. Bearing in mind that delirium and fainting were also perceived as related phenomena, it is safe to argue that the three exemplars of impaired consciousness were perceived by these Hippocratic doctors – just as we do nowadays – as a group of medical conditions that shared some common clinical features (hence our methodological choice is not an artificial anachronic modern imposition on the ancient material).[25]

Levels of consciousness

In line with the idea of a link between the three exemplars, it could be argued that the deepest and the most superficial depths of sleep – that is, the extremes of this spectrum – are, precisely, at the blurry borders where this prototype starts to blend with the

---

[23] *Epid. VII. CUF 108*, 2: 111, 14–15.

[24] ἐντὸς ἑωυτοῦ ἐγένετο ('being in his mind') is also used to talk about recovery from both a delirious sleep (*Epid. VII. CUF 2, 4*: 49, 21) and fainting (*Epid. VII. CUF 1, 7*: 48, 20).

[25] The idea of the disruption of senses as the common ground for all three prototypes of impaired consciousness – although intuited by the Hippocratic authors, as shown in previous passages – is explicitly proposed by Aristotle. As Thumiger (2017: 299) rightly argues, he related sleep, delirium and fainting as conditions caused by the interruption of perception (*Somn. et Vig.* 455b4–6).

others (fainting and delirium, respectively). As we shall see, Hippocratic medical writers resorted to two main linguistic devices when attempting to describe these changing levels of consciousness (and they found a correspondence between them and the seriousness of the diseases).

The widest used mechanism was nuancing and qualifying the specific terms through adjectives, adverbs or descriptive periphrasis: the writer of the first catastasis of *Epidemics II* describes – while talking about skin rashes in summer – a parallel progression between disturbed sleep (that is, a change in the level of consciousness) and the peak of the disease. He starts by explaining how women were not stuporous before the onset of the condition, and once it had started, πρόσθεν δὲ οὐ κάρτα ἦσαν κωματώδεις … κωματώδεις δὲ καὶ ὑπνώδεις τὸ θέρος καὶ μέχρι Πληϊάδων δύσιος, ἔπειτα μὴν ἀγρυπνίαι μᾶλλον ('though stuporous and somnolent (*kômatôdeis*,[26] *hupnôdeis*) during the summer until the setting of the Pleiades, afterwards there were instead periods of sleeplessness (*agrupniai*)').[27] The clarification that *kôma* was *hupnôdes* during that summer is not irrelevant, because in other cases it can be slightly different. In fact, in the third catastasis of *Epidemics III*, patients affected with ardent fever and *phrenitis* suffered ἢ τὸ κῶμα συνεχές οὐχ ὑπνῶδες, ἢ μετὰ πόνων ἄγρυπνοι ('either continuous non-somnolent stupor (*kôma suneches ouch hupnôdes*), or sleeplessness with distress (*meta ponôn agrupnoi*)').[28] Note the writer's exquisite precision when separating the non-somnolent continuous stupor from sleepless restlessness with discomfort.

On other occasions doctors are less sophisticated and make do with simple adjectives. Certain severely ill patients who were stuporous (*kômatôdees*), ἢ βαρὺ κῶμα παρείπετο ἢ μικροὺς καὶ λεπτοὺς ὕπνους κομᾶσθαι ('either suffered a deep stupor (*baru kôma*), or had light and short snatches of sleep (*leptous hupnous*)').[29] Similarly, the

---

[26] The notion of *kôma* refers to some kind of sleep disturbance with impaired consciousness, as McDonald (2009a: 42) suggests.
[27] *Epid. II. LCL 3, 1*: 44, 26; 45, 1–4. As McDonald (2009a: 41) has accurately pointed out, *agrupnia* designates a state of disturbed sleep and restlessness, probably accompanied by mental or physical discomfort.
[28] *Epid. III. CUF* catastasis VI.2: 84, 6–7.   [29] *Epid. III. CUF* catastasis XI.2: 88, 4–5.

author of *Prorrhetic I* states that κωματώδεες νωθροὶ οὐ πάνυ παρὰ αὐτοῖσιν ('patients affected with heavy stupor (*kômatôdees nôthroi*) are not well in their senses').[30]

In all these cases, changes in the level of consciousness seem to be correlated with clinical worsening of the patient. Particularly explicit of this parallel progression between severity of disease and depth of sleep is the case of Python's child: ὁ πυρετὸς παρωξύνετο, καὶ ἡ καταφορὴ διὰ τῶν αὐτῶν . . . αὐτίκα τὸ κῶμα ἐπέπαυτο, καὶ ὁ πυρετὸς ἐπεπρήϋντο ('the fever peaked and so did drowsiness (*kataphorê*) to the same extent (*dia tôn autôn*)'). This doctor does not seem to distinguish between *kataphorê* and *kôma*, because after the treatment he states that 'immediately drowsiness (*kôma*) stopped, and the fever became mild'.[31] Possibly this is a case of partial synonymy, which will be discussed later.

The other linguistic device to grade the depths of sleep, which was also common in modern times before the emergence of the GCS, is the use of diminishing suffixes.[32] Probably, the alteration of consciousness that the wife of Dromeades suffered on the fourth day after the onset of symptoms, *hupekarôthê*,[33] was slightly less than she would have had, had she been hit in the temples: πληγαὶ καίριοι καὶ καροῦσαι αἱ κροταφίτιδες γίνονται ('blows to the temples are mortal and cause stupor (*karousai*)').[34] Similarly, in *Prorrhetic I* (*LCL 38*) the writer claims that *hupagrupniê* is associated with diarrhoea. This prefixed derivation to grade levels of consciousness extends also to the syndromes related to hyperactive impaired consciousness (Theodorous' wife *elêrei* and *hupelêrei* alternately, *Epid. VII. CUF 25.2*: 13; 3, 19).

It appears that these linguistic devices evidence an explicit effort among these doctors to study various and changeable degrees of disconnection from the environment, which paralleled the degree of compromise of their patients. Within the spectrum of consciousness, drowsiness, agitated sleep and wakeful hypoactive delirium, on the one hand, and deep unreactive states of disconnection and fainting,

[30] *Prorrh. I. LCL 37*: 176, 23–4.
[31] *Epid. VII. CUF 118.2*: 114, 19–20; *118.3*: 115, 3–4.
[32] Comatous and hypocomatous were common terms to describe the level of consciousness before they could be quantitatively defined by the GCS.
[33] *Epid. I. CUF A11, XXVII.11*: 56, 10.   [34] *Artic. LCL 30*: 252, 21–2.

on the other, seem to both be in the peripheries of normal dormancy, just outside the limits of healthy sleep. Moreover, the more the clinical presentations differ from the ideal prototype of dreamless quiet sleep, the sicker the patient.

Terminology, mental capacities or HOFs, and the idea of mind

Terminology to describe the peripheries of sleep

Ever since Galen, scholars have tried to understand the exact meaning of the Hippocratic 'vocabulary of insanity'.[35] A usual strategy in recent studies has been to link the specific terms to the verbs and abstract nouns from which they derive. Thus, diseases like *phrenitis* or symptoms like *paraphronêsis* and *ekphrones* were related to the verb *phroneô* ('to think' or 'to be sound') and its more abstract derived noun *phronêsis*.[36] Similarly, *paranoia, paranoeô, paranoos*, to an abnormal way of performing the verb *noeô* ('to reason') and its abstract construct *nous*, contrary to their sound and healthy opposite, *katanoeô*. The same could be claimed about *suniêmi* ('to understand', 'to comprehend'), *sunesis* and their disturbed derivatives *parasunesis, asunetos*.[37] I consider this quest for a strict definition and delimitation of each term to be futile.

If we turn to our current technical language for such issues, there is no clear distinction between 'delirium', 'derangement', 'confusion' and 'disorientation'. In fact, two doctors presented with the same case would not necessarily choose exactly the same term to describe it, because these words have fuzzy edges. The very nature of the phenomenon is characterised by constant fluctuations, which make it difficult to choose only one of these categories.[38] Even if the terms do have subtle semantic differences, in actual clinical practice, they tend to be used

---

[35] The most important analyses on this topic are di Benedetto's (1986: 43–7), Pigeaud's (1987: 15–19) and Thumiger's (2013: 63–81). All three scholars focus on the composition of terms, the exact meaning of suffixes and lexemes, or they compare the collocations with older or contemporary extant sources. Other scholars have strived to seek equivalent modern translations (Matentzoglu, 2011: 7).

[36] Thumiger (2013: 69).   [37] Thumiger (2013: 75–6).

[38] Josephson and Miller (2018: 24).

interchangeably.[39] In other words, our clinical vocabulary disproves Langslow's postulate that unlike everyday language, where synonymy is mostly partial, in technical language synonyms are always absolute.[40] On the contrary, our medical vocabulary for impaired consciousness is mainly comprised of partial synonyms.

I have already highlighted this phenomenon when analysing the case studies in Part I (where different delirium terms such as *parakruô, parakoptô, paraphroneô*, etc. – some hyperactive and some hypoactive – were used interchangeably). I therefore do not agree with Thumiger's claim that ancient terms are interchangeable in modern translations because the subtleties are inaccessible for modern readers.[41] I propose, instead, that they were also interchangeable among ancient doctors, and it could even be argued that the phenomenon is not limited to the vocabulary of wakeful impaired consciousness. We have just seen how it is also extensive in sleeping terminology, where *kataphorê* and *kôma* are both associated with drowsy impaired consciousness and used as partial synonyms (in Python's child's account),[42] whereas *agrupniê* tends to suggest a more agitated sleep.

In terms of the historical debate about the intellectual context, this vocabulary bears testimony to a certain regularity or a certain community of ideas within the diversity of the HC. This specialised terminology seems to share several common features and to be in a developed stage of evolution: the abundance of verbs,[43] the extensive coinage of terms by derivation[44] and the repeated use of certain prefixes show both that doctors felt familiar with these terms and that they had similar ways of thinking and making sense of the world through language. In other words, the symmetries in the way that terms are coined and used may be reflecting a converging relationship between thought and expression of new ideas among these medical writers.[45] Therefore, the development of this jargon,

---

[39] The closest modern doctors can get to a distinction between these terms is whether they point towards hypoactive disturbance, such as 'stupor', or conversely, towards impaired consciousness with hyperactive responsiveness, such as 'agitation' (Josephson and Miller, 2018: 24).

[40] Langslow (2000: 21).   [41] Thumiger (2013: 82).

[42] *Epid. VII. CUF 118.2*: 114, 19–20; *118.3*: 115, 3–4.   [43] Langslow (2000: 23–4).

[44] Lloyd (1983: 158).   [45] Cross (2018: 12).

which enabled them to articulate relevant nuances for their novel theories, can be thought of as another sign of these physicians' distinction as a group and their claim to authority ahead of competing opponents.

In a nutshell, the terminology to describe delirium, sleep and its peripheries seems to refer to changeable conditions that can acquire opposing types of symptoms. A group of similar terms is used to describe states of utter bewilderment and passivity in the peripheries of sleep, on the one hand, and hyperactive impaired consciousness and hallucinations, on the other. The fact that, despite such contrasting presentations, the authors used equivalent terms constitutes a strong hint that they regarded them as essentially similar illnesses or as different manifestations of the same condition. When collating the collocations and the descriptions of these terms throughout the different authors, treatises and conditions, there seems to be a certain interchangeability and affinity in the meaning, which reminds us of the partial synonymy in our own vocabulary for impaired consciousness.[46] Undoubtedly, in a delirious person signs and symptoms are in constant change and fluctuation: within one single episode, one can be sleeping, agitated, drowsy, talking nonsense or silently staring into the void. It is understandable, therefore, that the different terms accounted for all those findings in some texts, but for only some of them in others.

HOFs in the Hippocratic texts

Closely related to the above-commented terminology, there is a number of vague or ill-defined concepts that these authors considered to be relevant in discussions about impaired consciousness (the derivatives of which were used to describe delirious symptoms). Such concepts – *phronêsis*, *sunesis*, *nous* (among others) – seem to subsume various combinations of capacities that are nowadays included in our idea of consciousness, for example, perception, movement, speech and reasoning. In other

---

[46] There are also examples of partial synonymy in non-technical texts. In Aristophanes' *Clouds* (*Nu.* 844–6) *paraphronountos* is used interchangeably with *paranoias* and *manian*.

words, they loosely group together constructs that correspond to what we nowadays regard as HOFs.[47]

If we go back once again to the study cases discussed in Part I, for the author of *Diseases I* the hallucinatory and delirious component of *phrenitis* was caused by bile affecting the *sunesis*.[48] The same problem, according to another nosological treatise, *On affections* (*Aff. LCL*: 10), originated in a stricken *nous* (*tou nou parakoptei*), and yet another medical writer related hallucinations to the *gnômê* (an abstract derivative of the verb *gignôskô*, 'to know, to perceive').

The latter discussed this idea in a short work that explores the different physiological and pathological aspects of glands:

ἡ γνώμη ταράσσεται, καὶ περίεισιν ἀλλοῖα φρονέων, καὶ ἀλλοῖα ὁρέων· φέρων τὸ ἦθος τῆς νούσου σεσηρόσι μειδιήμασι καὶ ἀλλοκότοισι φαντάσμασιν. *Glan. 12.2. Brill(C.)*: 76, 18–18.

The *gnômê* is disturbed, and [the sufferers] end up both thinking and seeing aberrations – things that are different [from reality] – as they bear this disease with a grinning laughter and strange visions.

It is interesting to point out that the author perceives this phenomenon as being different from spasms (that is, movement disturbances), speechlessness and breathing difficulties, which he associates with a bewildered (*aphronei*) *nous* (*Glan. 12.2. Brill (C.)*: 76, 13–15) in cases of *apoplexy*.

It seems that *gnômê*, *sunesis*, *nous* (and also *phronêsis* and *dianoia*) were associated according to these doctors with different combinations of HOFs, which played an important role in the workings of the mind, and therefore were involved in the development of impaired consciousness when affected.

[47] Alongside these terms, there are other constructs, mainly *thumos* and *psuchê* (that we often equate with philosophical representations of the soul and the spirit), which in certain passages are also related to these concepts: the author of *On diseases of girls* associated the *thumos* with hallucinations (*Virg. CUF II.3*: 190, 4–8), and the author of *On breaths* linked the alterations of consciousness during drunkenness with changes in the *psuchai* and the *phronemata* located in it (*Flat. CUF 14.3*: 122, 6–10).
In the next part I will discuss the idea of the soul that emerges from the analysis of impaired consciousness, and suggest that *psuchê* (and *thumos* to a lesser degree) is more usually conceived as a broader concept that often operates above the level of mental capacities, and can be determinant of the boundary between life and death.
[48] φρενῖτις δ' οὕτως ἔχει· τὸ αἷμα ἐν τῷ ἀνθρώπῳ πλεῖστον συμβάλλεται μέρος συνέσιος·...
(*Morb. I.30. LCL*: 158, 1–2).

In order to elucidate the way in which Hippocratic authors conceived, organised and subsumed the cognitive capacities, it is worth highlighting three outstanding features of these constructs: the divorce between the etymological stems of these terms and the vocabulary used in the clinical descriptions; their blurred boundaries, in other words, the vagueness and the overlapping of notions within each concept; and finally, the linguistic (non-etymological) connection between these theoretical ideas and the actual clinical manifestations.

Lack of etymological link between symptoms and these HOFs-constructs[49]

The futility of an etymological analysis becomes evident in any description where some of the above-mentioned concepts appear associated with symptoms.[50] To name but a few, the young virgins suffer *paranoia, paraphrosunê* and they *paraphroneoun*, yet the problem does not seem to be in their *nous* (etymologically related to *paranoia*) nor in their *phronêsis* (etymologically related to *paraphroneein*). On the contrary, the *thumos* is affected. Similarly, the author of *Diseases I* talks about *paranoeô-paranoia-paranooi ginontai*, and *paraphroneô*, but he associates these abnormalities with a disturbed *sunesis* (again, neither *nous* nor *phronêsis*). In this sense, one could even wonder whether *tou nou parakoptontos*, characteristic of *phrenitis* in *On affections* (10), can be equated with the above-mentioned *paranoia* of the *sunesis*, given that both writers are describing the same condition. It appears that the derived compounds utilised to talk about clinical manifestations have become estranged from their etymological roots.[51]

---

[49] I am not suggesting that one should expect etymology to explain the meaning or uses of the words. My approach presents an alternative solution to the one offered by the existing scholarship, which has mainly focused on the meaning of the composing elements of these terms (especially di Benedetto, 1986: 43–7; Pigeaud, 1987: 15–19; and Thumiger, 2013: 63–81).

[50] Craik (2015: 278–9).

[51] There is also an example of this etymological divorce in an extra-medical source. In a Euripidean fragment '[we, old men] have no nous, yet we believe we think correctly' (νοῦς δ' οὐκ ἔνεστιν, οἰόμεσθα δ' εὖ φρονεῖν (*Eur. fr. LCL*: 26, 4)), thereby suggesting a correlation between having a *nous* and being sane, or being able to think (*euphronein*).

Various combinations of mental capacities within the constructs

Another salient feature of these concepts is their lack of standardisation, which causes contradictions, overlapping and vagueness concerning which mental capacities are included within them. None of these concepts is clearly or consistently defined. Actually, their scope can vary even within a single treatise.[52]

Despite explicit attempts by the author of *On the sacred disease* to define *phronêsis*, some contradictions arise when analysing the treatise. Chapter 7[53] explains how the airflow that enters the brain enables *phronêsis* and 'the movement of the limbs' (*CUF 7. 4*: 15, 19–20), thereby distinguishing them as two separate capacities. Naturally, when the phlegm blocks the air, two consequences occur: on the one hand, due to the compromised *phronêsis* ἄφωνον καθιστᾶσι καὶ ἄφρονα τὸν ἄνθρωπον ('the person becomes dumb and senseless', which suggests that *phronêsis* subsumes intelligence or reasoning and perceptions;[54] on the other, the limbs suffer spasms and involuntary movements. Later on, chapter 16 reiterates the importance of air as the provider of *phronêsis* to the brain, but immediately afterwards it is stated:

οἱ δὲ ὀφθαλμοὶ καὶ τὰ ὦτα καὶ ἡ γλῶσσα καὶ αἱ χεῖρες καὶ οἱ πόδες οἷα ἂν ὁ ἐγκέφαλος γινώσκῃ, τοιαῦτα πρήσσουσι. γίνεται γὰρ ἐν ἅπαντι τῷ σώματι τῆς φρονήσιος, ὡς ἂν μετέχῃ τοῦ ἠέρος. *Morb. Sacr. CUF 16.2*: 29, 8–11.

Eyes, ears, tongue, hands and feet can accomplish however much the brain can discern. The body has its share of *phronêsis* in the same proportion as it has its share of air.

Unlike the previous definition, in this passage all the functions that are impaired during a seizure are considered as part of *phronêsis*, including perceptions, speech and the movement of the limbs. Yet again, in chapter 17 the author establishes a clear contrast between diaphragm (*phrenes*), heart and brain: whereas

---

[52] Thumiger (2017: 394) also observes the lack of stable semantic differentiation among these concepts.
[53] I follow the chapter division of the Budé edition (which in turn follows Littré's), as opposed to the Jones edition.
[54] *Morb. Sacr. CUF 7.5*: 15, 22.

the former two are able to perceive – ἡ καρδίη αἰσθάνεταί τε μάλιστα καὶ αἱ φρένες ('the heart and the diaphragm do indeed perceive')[55] – it is only the brain that partakes in *phronêsis* (*CUF 17.3*: 31, 7–8),[56] which suggests that perceptions are not part of what he includes within the notion. This example – even accepting the theory of different writers[57] – reveals the embryonic state of this terminology, insofar as words are clearly used with a technical intention but their usage is not standardised yet.[58] In this sense, I disagree with van der Eijk's translations of *phronêsis* as 'consciousness' and *sunesis* as 'understanding'.[59] We should regard these notions as rudimentary attempts to fragment what we nowadays include within the sphere of consciousness, but not as clearly defined and consistent concepts. As a matter of fact, things get even more complicated if we contrast these passages with the above-commented excerpt of *On glands*, in which the author fragments most of the same HOFs in a different manner and defines them as *gnômê* and *nous*.

Another ambiguous approach, where lack of standardisation manifests as overlapping of concepts, is offered in the highly philosophical treatise *On regimen*. This long and elaborate work addresses several topics under the general overarching premise that the human regimen has some influence over health.[60] As far as consciousness is concerned, its medical writer theorised about *gnômê*, *dianoia* (a compound of *nous*) and *phronêsis*. Although a priori they look like different concepts, their differences become sometimes blurred. Chapter 1, for example, opens by stating:

εἰ μέν μοί τις ἐδόκει τῶν πρότερον συγγραψάντων περὶ διαίτης ἀνθρωπίνης ... ὀρθῶς ἐγνωκὼς συγγεγραφέναι πάντα διὰ παντὸς ὅσα δυνατὸν ἀνθρωπίνῃ γνώμῃ περιληφθῆναι... *Vict. CMG 1.1*: 122, 1–3.

---

55 *Morb. Sacr. CUF 17.3*: 31, 6–7.
56 Jones (1923: 181, n. 2) has also pointed out the distinction between *aisthêsis* and *phronêsis*.
57 A debate about chapters 14–17 being later additions to the book is reported by Hüffmeier (1961: 51–2).
58 Langslow (2000: 13).
59 van der Eijk (2005: 127). For a larger discussion about the difficulty in translating the term *phronêsis*, see Thumiger (2017: 389–90).
60 Craik (2015: 270–1).

If it seemed to me that any of those who composed treatises about the human regimen ... had throughout composed them with correct knowledge (*orthôs egnôkôs*) about everything that the human *gnômê* can comprehend...[61]

By the end of this same chapter, however, the author claims that 'it is part of the same *dianoia* to know what was correctly said (*gnônai ta orthôs*) as well as to discover what was not [yet] said'.[62] The similar vocabulary connected to each term (*orthôs egnôkôs* and *gnônai ta orthôs*), along with the general sense of both statements, points towards notions that are similar. Further into the discussion, *dianoia* virtually disappears, *nous* is mentioned twice,[63] and the author claims that 'the invisible human *gnômê* enables one to cognise visible things',[64] as though this concept was an HOF related to perception. Nevertheless, by the end of the first book, in chapter 35, perception seems to depend on *phronêsis*, thereby producing, again, overlapping of the notions.[65]

It is worthwhile taking a closer look at this long and complex passage, which many scholars have tried to make sense of.[66] Unlike other occurrences, in this excerpt *phronêsis* is regarded as a condition or a state of the *psuchê*,[67] with a variable aspect (discussed in chapter 35) that has control over movements, perceptions, cognitive functioning (including our idea of intelligence) and emotions.[68]

---

[61] Of note in this passage is the rhetorical 'othering' of the previous writers (*tôn proteron sungrapsantôn*), which is an example of the intellectual debate that was taking place among these authors, in which they distanced themselves from other groups.

[62] τῆς αὐτῆς ἐστὶ διανοίης γνῶναι τὰ ὀρθῶς εἰρημένα, ἐξευρεῖν τε τὰ μήπω εἰρημένα (*Vict. CUF I.1*: 122, 18).

[63] Bartos (2015: 187).

[64] γνώμη ἀνθρώπου ἀφανὴς γινώσκουσα τὰ φανερά (*Vict. CMG I.12*: 136, 10–11).

[65] In *On the art*, *gnômê* enables mental acquaintance with imperceptible things. Just as the eyes facilitate sight, *gnômê* facilitates knowing (*Art. 2.1 Brill(M)*: 51, 19–20). As Mann (2012, 89–90) has accurately pointed out, *gnômê* is here independent of perception.

[66] Hüffmeier (1961: 68–82) analyses the value of *phronêsis* in *On regimen*, *On breaths* and *On the sacred disease*. Pigeaud (1987: 41–7) sees in this passage 'une théorie de la connaisance'. Hankinson (1991: 202–6) explores the relation psychology–physiology and reflects on the ways of thinking and theorising amongst the Hippocratic doctors. Lopez Morales (1999: 514–19) and Jouanna (2013: 100–3) have explored the connection between fire and water in this passage with bile and phlegm in *On the sacred disease*. The latter develops his hypothesis about two typologies of madness based on these texts. Lastly, Matentzoglu (2011: 72–9) and Byl (2002: 217–24) offer a systematic description of the classification.

[67] Hüffmeier (1961: 64–5) has made a distinction between *Zustand* (condition) and *Vermögen* (function, capacity), when discussing *On breaths*. I find this particularly useful in understanding this passage.

[68] Matentzoglu (2011: 72–9).

According to the account, the nature of the *phronêsis* depends on the proportion of moistness or dryness within the fire and water in the *psuchê*. It is conceived as a spectrum that ranges between *phronimôtaton* (*Vict. CMG 1.35*: 150, 30) and *aphronestaton* (*Vict. CMG 1.35*: 152, 7).[69] Indeed, the whole passage is meant to show how different mixtures of the two elements yield different levels of *phronêsis*, which manifest as various degrees of delirium, affective vulnerability, intelligence, perception and motility.[70] It is in this sense that I consider that the concept can be likened to consciousness and disagree with Bartos, who equates it only with intelligence.[71] Undoubtedly, when consciousness is impaired some or many of these capacities can be compromised, and the seven possible mixtures described in the passage refer to various combinations of deficiencies at each level of *phronêsis*. Therefore, it is arguably not only 'the physiology of thinking'[72] that this author is describing, but the physiology of consciousness more generally.

Inevitably, this reminds us of our current gradual understanding of consciousness through the GCS.[73] The reasoning underlying both systems is that a certain level of *phronêsis* or consciousness, respectively, corresponds to observable cognitive responses. Furthermore, the ancient doctor resorted to linguistic devices similar to the ones utilised by modern doctors when trying to describe progressive levels of impairment. The Hippocratic writer contrasts *maniê*, the most altered state of *phronêsis*, with a condition that can easily become *maniê* but has not reached it yet, defining it as *hupomainesthai* (*Vict. CMG 1.35*: 156, 4). In a similar manner, before the emergence of the numeric GCS, doctors used to talk about 'comatose' and 'sub-comatose' patients. The analogy not only highlights the gradual nature of the

---

[69] *Phronimotaton* is associated with the wettest fire and the driest water. Perhaps this idea is part of the above-mentioned tradition present in Aretaeus' link between dryness and clairvoyance during *kausôn*, and in Galen's discussion in *QAM* (*Teubner 4*: 42–3).

[70] Matentzoglu (2011: 72–9).   [71] Bartos (2015: 191–5).   [72] Bartos (2015: 199).

[73] The Glasgow Coma Scale comprises three components that are assessed separately: eye opening (E), verbal response (V) and best motor response (M). Each of these aspects is given a score that increases as the individual becomes more conscious. I have elsewhere discussed other medical scales in current use to assess delirium and cognition that also correlate certain clinical findings with a degree of compromise (Pelavski, 2020: 11–12). Therefore, all these contemporary tools use a similar principle as the one that this author is suggesting to measure the soundness of related capacities.

impairment in mental capacities (similar to the linguistic devices used to describe the different depths of sleep), but it also shows the need to quantify it, which doctors from such different worlds both felt in their actual practice. Additionally, it illustrates what Langslow has called 'the preference of technical languages for certain forms of derivation'.[74]

To be sure, the collocations and scope of all these terms reveal that they were in the process of becoming specialised vocabulary.[75] As Cross explains, 'written prose most closely reflects the everyday conversational exchanges'.[76] Hence, sometimes they were used as technical terms, whereas on other occasions they appear to be non-specialised words. Like the above-discussed terminology to describe symptoms, this is another example of the emergence of prose as a means for Hippocratic authors to express new shared ideas (although, as the variation in meaning seems to suggest, in a lower stage of development).

Finally, there are other examples that not only illustrate the faint boundaries between these constructs, but also further reinforce the hypothesis about fuzzy edges between sleep and wakeful impaired consciousness. While in *On breaths* (*CUF 14*), sleep affected *phronêsis*, in *Epidemics VI* (*LCL 8.5*: 262), it disturbs (*tarassetai*) the *gnômê*, and in *On regimen* (*Vict. CMG 4.86*) it is a state of the *psuchê*. This could explain why delirium and sleep were sometimes clinically difficult to distinguish for these doctors: because they were explained through the alteration of related theoretical constructs. Or put in another way, these constructs that became altered during delirium and sleep can be framed as embryonic ideas of consciousness. As Thumiger has remarked, we can currently divide this tangle of ideas, concepts and capacities into more specific intellective functions (she distinguishes seven).[77] Even if some of them would not be nowadays considered to strictly belong within our definition of consciousness, they all become impaired in conditions that affect it.

---

[74] Langslow (2000: 24). In this case moderns and ancients have chosen equivalent prefixes.
[75] Their lack of standardisation is evidenced by the fact that they either used the same name to designate two or more concepts, or conversely, alternative names to designate the same or very similar notions (Lloyd, 1983: 160).
[76] Cross (2018: 12).   [77] Thumiger (2017: 394–5).

Therefore, it is useful to roughly frame these ancient concepts as rudimentary constructs of consciousness.

Phrasal terms: the linguistic link between clinical findings and theoretical constructs

Given the lack of an etymological correspondence between these sets of HOFs and the partial synonyms used to describe the symptoms of delirium, the last point that I aim to address is a plausible hypothesis about their correlation: despite this divorce, there is a clinical link between them. In order to understand this connection, it is useful to look at what Langslow has called 'phrasal terms'.[78] These are lexicalised phrases that have the status of a technical term. The corpus abounds in such constructions that are comprised of a noun head, which – in our case – is abstract and can be assimilated to one of these constructs subsuming HOFs, and different kinds of determiners. A few examples are *gnômês paraphoroi* – 'delirious *gnômê*' (*Coac. LCL 31*: 12, 22), *gnômê kataplêx* – 'stricken *gnômê*' (*Mul. II. LCL 92*: 424, 15), *tên gnômên blabentes* – 'confused, distracted *gnômê*' (*Acut. CUF 17.1*: 2–3) and *ekplêxies tês gnômês* – 'disturbances of the *gnômê*' (*Aer. CUF 23.3*: 243, 5). Or even with other heads: *dianoia thrasuterê* – 'a more insolent *dianoia*' (*Epid. VII. CUF 1.6*: 48, 12), *tou nou parakoptei* – 'the *nous* is deranged' (*Aff. LCL 10*: 18, 9), *parallaxies phrenôn* – 'aberration of the *phrênes*' (*Acut. Sp. LCL 1*: 262, 12).[79] Common to all these instances is the metaphorical dimension of the determiner:[80] the nouns are abstract theoretical constructions, which the authors metaphorically linked to determiners that convey the idea of compromise, deviation or blow. Considering that these phrases are lexicalisations and bearing in mind the 'shorthand nature' of many compositions,[81] we can hypothesise that the verbs used in isolation (such as *parapherô*,

---

[78] Langslow (2000: 206–68) claims that phrasal terms can be considered as a specific subcategory within the 'stehende Redewendungen' or stock phrases described by Hellweg (1985: 29–52).

[79] Euripides introduces another of them in his *Hippolytus*: *parakoptei phrenas* (*Hipp.* 238).

[80] Langslow (2000: 178).

[81] According to van der Eijk (1997: 104–6) many syntactic peculiarities in the HC can be explained by assuming that the compositions were 'a kind of shorthand for private use or circulation among specialists' intelligible only to the writer or his colleagues.

parakrouô) evolved from previously lexicalised phrasal terms that lost their head through metonymy or brachylogy. In most cases, we cannot be sure whether the author was thinking of the *gnômê*, *phronêsis*, *nous* or any other of the abstract theoretical concepts into which the ancient authors subsumed the HOFs, but at least we can posit that an embryonic idea of consciousness was perceived as being compromised. In this respect, I disagree with Thumiger; I think that these abstract constructs (presupposed in the noun head, even when it was omitted) were often treated like concrete body parts, in the sense that they could suffer and be affected by disease.[82]

In summary, the analysis suggests that the Hippocratic doctors did attempt to break down the abstract notion of consciousness into smaller HOFs, which they variously grouped into discrete concepts. These passages demonstrate that terminology to discuss HOFs was not fully developed, nor was the theoretical framework by which doctors understood these medical conditions. In this respect, Lloyd has accurately pointed out – while discussing Greek anatomical vocabulary – that the oscillation in the meaning of technical terms often indicates the backward state of theoretical speculation.[83] As a matter of fact, even now, scientific journals acknowledge the confusion and overlapping of concepts in the semantic field of consciousness ('awareness', 'wakefulness', 'perception', 'vigilance').[84]

On a more theoretical level, the analysis supports the idea that delirium and sleep were often linked – in these doctors' conception – to the impairment of what we could designate as an embryonic notion of consciousness. It is also in this regard that we can find a sense of consistency and unity across different authors and treatises within the HC.

---

[82] Thumiger (2017: 398).   [83] Lloyd (1983: 153).   [84] Sanders et al. (2012: 946).

CHAPTER 9

SLEEP IN POST-HELLENISTIC SOURCES

The landscape slightly changed in the post-Hellenistic treatises due to the emergence of *lethargy* as a specific sleeping disease. It could be argued that the authors maintained the key elements of discussion that were apparent in the Hippocratic corpus, but they reformulated them. As a result, we are still able to find ambiguities and tensions between health and disease, consciousness and unconsciousness, as well as a redefinition of the kind of disconnection that characterised sleep, where the accounts are shaped by the particular interests and the specific methodological approach of each author.

Disconnection during sleep

The status of sleep in Celsus' *On medicine* has some parallels with the Hippocratic corpus,[1] but it also has divergences. Indeed, the topic offers a good example of the author's encyclopaedic approach, in which he makes different sources compatible by juxtaposing some coincidences and some discrepancies without evident contradictions. In this sense, Celsus maintains the characterisation of sleep as a disconnection from the environment; however, his idea of disconnection is much stronger. According to his view, individuals are not only insensitive to the world surrounding them while asleep, but they also seem to be unaware of their own bodily sensations.

The former and more Hippocratic type of disconnection is evidenced by the repeated insistence on applying physical stimuli to patients with *lethargy*: *aegros ... excitare, expergiscatur aeger* (*Med. 3.20*: 1, 2). Such prodding constitutes an active attempt at reconnecting them with outside reality through external agents aimed at waking them up, such as strong unpleasant odours, or by provoking sneezing.

---

[1] Martinez (1974: 68).

On the other hand, the interruption of one's own perception during sleep, which is a more radical (and un-Hippocratic) kind of disconnection, is illustrated by the use of *anodyna* ... *quae somno dolorem levant* ('painkilling [drugs] that relieve pain through sleep').[2] Undoubtedly, such an idea is not compatible with the *psuchê* in full control of its household while sleeping (*Vict. CMG 4.86*),[3] even less so with the description of the patient who was so in touch with his perceptions that he enacted his own dreams while having them, and was afterwards capable of giving a full account of his vivid nightmares (*Int. LCL 48*). As will be discussed below, this complete disconnection from the environment as well as from the body as described by Celsus will make it easier for him to relate sleep to total loss of consciousness.

Aretaeus' take on this issue is evident in his discussion of *lethargy*, but he only adheres to the Hippocratic kind of disconnection. He considers that the patient is unaware of his environment because αἱ αἰσθήσιες πλέαι γίγνονται ἀτμῶν ('perceptions are full of vapours').[4] To cure the condition he also recommends – like Celsus – strong stimuli to wake sufferers up: ἐμβόησις· νουθεσίη ὀργίλη· δεῖμα ἐφ'οἷσι δειμαίνει ('shouts, angry reprimands and violent threats').[5] Unlike Celsus, though, he does not seem to support the radical disconnection described in *On medicine*. Sleep does not prevent individuals from feeling pain, which suggests that they do not become disconnected from their own bodily sensations. There is proof of this in the treatment for kidney lithiasis. There, Aretaeus explains that once the urinary stone falls into the bladder, ἄπονοί τε γίγνονται, οὐδ' ὄναρ δοκέειν τοῦ πόνου εἰθισμένοι ('they become free from pain, so that not even in their dreams do they consider themselves to be in pain'), which hints that they could potentially feel pain while asleep.[6]

---

[2] *Med. 5.25*: 1.
[3] I agree with Bartos' (2015: 202) interpretation of *On regimen*, that body and soul are still closely cooperating during sleep, even if the latter is more independent than during wakefulness.
[4] *CA I.2. CMG (H).V*: 99, 11.   [5] *CA I.2. CMG (H).V*: 98, 11–12.
[6] *CA II.8. CMG (H).VI*: 138, 16–17.

Fuzzy edges, clear boundaries and peripheries: sleep–wakefulness, health–disease

Regarding the ambiguities around sleep, both these authors seem to have negotiated their positions in respect to their Hippocratic predecessors and their more contemporary sources.

The boundaries of consciousness: ways of being conscious and unconscious

The distinction between sleep and wakeful impaired consciousness appears to have been a well-worn debate in the post-Hellenistic era. Despite Aristotle's statement that ἐνδέχεται γὰρ τοῦ ἐγρηγορέναι καὶ καθεύδειν ἁπλῶς θατέρου ὑπάρχοντος θάτερόν πῃ ὑπάρχειν ('although wakefulness and sleep exist separately from each other, it is possible for both to somehow coexist'),[7] medical writers struggled to identify these intermediate states. Such is the case of Caelius Aurelianus' version of Soranus,[8] who criticised Asclepiades for confusing sleep (*somno*) with stupor (*pressura*) caused by poppies:

his nos respondebimus differre pressuram a somno. contra naturam etenim pressura intelligitur, secundum naturam somnus. papavera autem pressuram, non somnum faciunt. *Aur. Acut. I.17*: 10, 22–5.

To him [to Asclepiades] we will reply that subduing differs from sleep, for the former is contrary to nature, whereas the latter is in accordance with nature. That is, the poppy subdues a person but it does not cause him to sleep.

In Celsus' account, painkillers offer a good example of the above discussion. Like Asclepiades (and unlike Soranus/Caelius Aurelianus), Celsus does not seem to have distinguished this nuance. He related the poppy (*papaver*) to *somnus*,[9] thereby equating sleep with the hypoactive type of impaired consciousness that a compound

---

[7] *Insomn. LCL 462.a.*

[8] Although Caelius Aurelianus is a much later author (around the fifth century CE), in the work referred to he was translating a treatise by Soranus, who did live between the end of the first and beginning of the second century CE (therefore, roughly contemporary with Aretaeus).

[9] Still referring to the *anodyna* pills (that calmed pain through sleep), Celsus adds: *potest tamen etiam ad conquendum, quod habet papaveris lacrimae* ('there is, however, one that helps digestion, which is composed of poppy-tears', *Med. 5.25*: I).

containing poppy would likely have caused. However, he did clearly differentiate sleep from hyperactive delirium. His definition of *lethargy* in opposition to *phrenesis* illustrates this: *in eo difficilior somnus, prompta ad omnem audaciam mens est: in hoc marcor et inexpugnabililis paene dormiendi necessitas* ('In [*phrenesis*] sleeping is difficult, and the mind is inclined to any kind of insolence. In [*lethargy*] there is drowsiness (*marcor*)[10] and a hardly bearable need to sleep').[11]

As a matter of fact, Celsus seems to have almost conceived sleep as an all-or-nothing phenomenon. Such a simplification might explain why *On medicine* leaves out a few conditions mentioned in other post-Hellenistic sources, where the boundaries between wakeful hallucinations, drowsy deliriums and nightmares were faint. *Catalepsia* or *catochos* and *tuphomania*, which are discussed in the pseudo-Galenic *Medical definitions*,[12] are not mentioned in his encyclopaedia. Furthermore, he even ignored the cognitive symptoms that other authors assimilated to *lethargy*, thereby further distancing sleep from conscious mental processing.[13]

---

[10] Although *marcor* can also refer to putrefaction, no other sources hint at such a phenomenon. Conversely, Celsus' description seems to be following a well-established tradition. Both the *Medical definitions* and the *Introduction* offer similar ideas: καταφορὰ δυσδιέγερτος ('drowsiness, difficulty in waking up', *Def. Med. 235. K. XIX*: 413, 4) and καταφορὰ γάρ ἐστι βαθεῖα καὶ δυσανάκλιτος ('drowsiness is deep, and it is difficult to get out of bed', *Introd. CUF XIII.25*: 57, 23).

[11] *Med. 3.20, 1*.

[12] εἴδη δὲ κατόχου τρία. ὁ μὲν γὰρ ὑπνώδης ὃς παράκειται τῷ ληθάργῳ. ὁ δὲ ἕτερος ἐγρηγορώς, ᾧ παράκειται τέτανος ... τρίτον εἶδος κατόχου ... γίνεται δὲ ἐκ μίγματος δύο ἀρρωστημάτων κατόχου τε καὶ φρενίτιδος ὥσπερ καὶ ἡ τυφομανία ('*Catalepsia* has three forms; the somnolent one that is similar to lethargy; the other one is wakeful, which resembles tetanus ... the third form of *catalepsia* ... is produced by the mixture of two illnesses, both *catalepsia* and *phrenitis*, in the same way as *tuphomania* as well', *Def. Med. 241. K.XIX*: 414, 15–18; 415, 1–3).
τυφομανία ἐστὶ λήθαργος παρακοπτικὸς ἢ παρακοπὴ ληθαργική. ἢ οὕτως τυφομανία ἐστὶ μικτὸν ἐκ φρενίτιδος καὶ ληθάργου πάθημα ('*Tuphomania* is a delirious lethargy, or a lethargic delirium. Otherwise, *tuphomania* is a mixture of *phrenitis* and *lethargy*', *Def. Med. 243. K.XIX*: 415, 7–9). Both definitions refer to diseases in the middle of the spectrum of consciousness.

[13] A few extant Hellenistic descriptions of *lethargy* include forgetfulness and delirium as important symptoms. The author of the *Introduction* states that affected individuals ἐπιλανθανόμενοι πάντων ὅσα λέγουσι ('forget about everything they say', *Introd. CUF XIII.25*: 57, 24). The *Anonymus Parisinus* mentions speech difficulties and a delirious dianoia (παραπαίουσι τῇ διανοίᾳ, *Anon. Paris. II.2*, 2: 12, 7).

This lack of fuzzy edges between hallucinations and nightmares (present in most other authors) is replicated in the terminology. Unlike the Hippocratic treatises, there is no overlap in Celsus' use of vocabulary: both falling asleep (*dormire, somnus accedere/ capere, soporare*, etc.) and waking up or being awake (*vigilare, excitare, expergisci*, etc.) are expressed with a lexicon that is only used in relation to sleep, and completely different from the terms used in descriptions of wakeful impaired consciousness and its recovery.

On the other hand, Celsus did seem to recognise a certain similarity between swoons and sleep. Although he did not elaborate on the activity of the *anima* during sleep – and this is why it seems to be independent of the soul in a superficial analysis – sleeping is perceived as a phenomenon akin to total loss of consciousness (with a link that is mainly based on the clinical presentation, rather than on a physiological explanation).[14]

Despite this asymmetry, where delirium seems to be totally unrelated to sleep as opposed to fainting, the explicit contrasts that Celsus makes between *phrenesis, lethargy* and *cardiacum* supports the hypothesis that the three ideal exemplars of impaired consciousness were somehow related in his understanding (and are not a mere modern idea forced onto his text), particularly considering that *phrenesis* was one among three possible presentations of *insania*, yet the only one worth explicitly opposing to the other prototypical presentations of impaired consciousness (*cardiacum* and *lethargy*).[15] This suggests that the second and third forms of *insania* (which we would now consider as mental illness) were so unrelated to impaired consciousness that they did not even need to be contrasted.

---

[14] I will later question this view and suggest that Celsus did have an idea of the soul involved in the process of sleep.

[15] A similar need for distinction appears in another post-Hellenistic text. The *Introduction* offers a Stoic-informed differentiation of the same selection of three entities: τῶν δὲ πνευμάτων μήτε ἐπιτεινομένων ἄγαν ὡς ἐπὶ τῶν φρενιτικῶν, μήτε ἐκλυομένων, ὡς ἐπὶ τῶν ληθαργικῶν, ἢ ἐπὶ τῶν ἐν καρδιακῇ διαθέσει ὄντων ('The *pneumata* are neither too tense as in *phrenitis*, nor too loose as in *lethargy*, or as in the *cardiac* condition', *Int. CUF* 13.3: 46, 20–3). Note how – despite grouping the three of them as comparable entities, much like Celsus, this author also draws a slight asymmetry between *phrenitis*, on the one hand, and *lethargy* and *cardiacum*, on the other.

Aretaeus also construed *phrenitis* and *lethargy* as opposed conditions; however, his eclectic method did not prevent him from equating sleep with hyperactive impaired consciousness. Evidence for this conception is given in the discussion on *pleuritis*: γίγνονται δὲ παράληροι· ἔστι δ᾽ ὅτε καὶ κωματώδεες, καὶ ἐν τῇ καταφορῇ παράφοροι ('[patients] become delirious (*paralêroi*); on occasion even stuporous (*kômatôdees*), and in their drowsiness (*kataphorê*) they are deranged (*paraphoroi*)').[16] This passage illustrates rather explicitly the way in which drowsiness and delirium may become one and the same phenomenon. Also, during certain acute exacerbations of *melancholia*, patients seem to suffer from threatening nightmares that are hard to distinguish from reality:

κατηφέες, νωθροὶ ἔασι ἀλόγως . . . ἄγρυπνοι, ἐκ τῶν ὕπνων ἐκθορυβούμενοι. ἔχει δὲ αὐτέους καὶ τάρβος ἔκτοπον, ἢν ἐς αὔξησιν τὸ νόσημα φοιτῇ, εὖτε καὶ ὄνειροι ἀληθέες, δειματώδεες, ἐναργέες. ὁκόσα γὰρ ὑπερεκτρέπονται οὔπω οἱ κακοῦ, τάδε ἐνύπνιον ὀρέουσι ὥρμησε. *SD I.5. CMG (H).III*: 40, 15–20.

With drowsy sunken eyes [sufferers] become irrational . . . [moreover, they are] restless and disturbed from their sleep. If the disease progresses, they are dominated by unjustified terror as well as true-looking, threatening and vivid dreams. Indeed, they are scared because they can see in their dreams the things that horrify them the most (even though they are actually not under threat).

The passage, indeed, reminds us of certain elements present in Hippocratic descriptions of hallucinations and visions (*Int. LCL 48*, and *Virg. CUF I.1*). In this description, however, the uncertain limit between sleep and wakefulness enables Aretaeus to reflect upon one of his constant concerns, which is the truth behind real-looking apparitions (in this case, visions in dreams come under scrutiny). In other words, not only the *phantasiai* of delirious *phrenitics* (as commented above), but also the *oneiroi alêthees* and the *enupnion* of the drowsy *melancholics*, question the relationship between perception and reality.[17]

---

[16] *SA I.9. CMG (H).I*: 12, 28–9.

[17] Such deliberations are also underpinned by powerful cultural constructions. As Aubert and White (1959: 48) have remarked, the idea that waking life is real life and the world of dreams is unreal is valid in our society but not necessarily in others (they give the example of the Ashanti, who can be punished for transgressing social rules in their dreams).

We can posit, therefore, that these lax boundaries between wakeful and drowsy impaired consciousness – added to the overlap between fainting and sleeping – suggest that Aretaeus also perceived our three prototypes of impaired consciousness to be related.[18] Furthermore, we can even find hints of a more theoretical relation between swoons, sleep and delirium in Aretaeus' pathophysiological explanations (apart from the clinical similarities just referred to).

There is an emphasis on the loss of heat during swoons (referred to as *thermê*[19] and *aleê tês zoês*[20]), which evokes the *psuxis emphutos*[21] of *lethargic* patients and opposes the alterations in the *oikeiou thalpeos*[22] during *phrenitis*. Ultimately, the distortion of any kind of heat, which was at the very boundary between life and death, also seems to cause some compromise of cognition, thereby unifying these three alterations of consciousness. In the context of Aretaeus' eclectic method, this could be interpreted as an example of *symphorêsis* (or, to put it more simply, a lax use of terminology).

In terms of Aretaeus' keen interest in perceptions, we have seen that an altered *aisthêsis* had a central place in the descriptions of delirium. The fact that in *lethargy* αἱ αἰσθήσεις πλέαι γίγνονται ἀτμῶν ('perceptions are full of vapours'),[23] and that they are also mentioned in relation to swoons (*SD I.7. CMG (H).III*: 44, 20 and *CD I.5. CMG (H).VII*: 156, 7), only confirms their key role in consciousness, and that they are a further trait that is shared by the three prototypical presentations.

To sum up, the way in which these authors conceive the limits between different forms of impaired consciousness and sleep mirrors their understanding of the boundaries between consciousness and unconsciousness. While Celsus conceives a clear-cut separation between wakeful impairment of cognitive capacities and sleep, and a certain continuity between the latter and hypoactive impaired consciousness, Aretaeus' take is more

---

[18] The blurred boundaries between sleep and total loss of consciousness will be discussed in detail when addressing the treatment of *saturiasis*.
[19] *CA I.10. CMG (H).V*: 114, 5–6.   [20] *CA I.4. CMG (H).V*: 103, 1–2.
[21] *CA I.2. CMG (H).V*: 98, 9.   [22] *CA I. CMG (H).V.1*: 96, 29.
[23] *CA I.2. CMG (H).V*: 99, 11.

in harmony with Hippocratic ideas. Like his Hippocratic predecessors, he understood such limits to be rather blurred, with
intermediate states between wakefulness, sleep and hypoactive
impaired consciousness. Moreover, although both post-
Hellenistic authors found links between the three exemplars, it
could be argued that Celsus' were mainly based on their similar
clinical features, whereas in Aretaeus (and also in the
Introduction) the connection was not only clinical, but also
pathophysiological.

Boundaries between health and disease

Despite this discrepancy concerning the nature of sleep and its
relation to wakefulness, Celsus and Aretaeus both seem to agree
with their Hippocratic predecessors about the liminal zone between
health and disease that the process occupies.

In the case of Celsus, this feature is illustrated in book 2, which
offers a good example of his encyclopaedic prowess. In a passage
that is virtually a translation from the HC, he is able to combine
both Hippocratic and un-Hippocratic ideas.

... gravis morbi periculum est ... ubi nocturna vigilia premitur, etiamsi interdiu
somnus accedit; ex quo tamen peior est, qui inter quartam horam et noctem est,
quam qui matutino tempore ad quartam. pessimum tamen est si somnus neque
noctu neque interdiu accedit: id enim fere sine continuo dolore esse non potest.
Neque vero signum bonum est etiam somno ultra debitum urgueri, peiusque, quo
magis se sopor interdiu noctuque continuat. *Med. 2.4:* 1–2.

There is danger of severe illness ... when [the patient] is worn out by
nocturnal wakefulness, even if during the daytime he gets some sleep. In
the latter case, however, it is worse to sleep between the fourth hour and
night-time, than between the morning hours and the fourth. Worst of all,
though, is if sleep comes neither during the night nor during the day, for
this can hardly ever happen without continuous pain. But it is not a good sign
either to be oppressed by sleep beyond measure, and the more the stupor
persists day and night, the worse it is.

This is part of a discussion on bad signs in illnesses and the text
follows almost word by word *Prognosis CUF 10*. However, Celsus
omits to mention the very last words, where μὴ κοιμᾶσθαι, μήτε τῆς
νυκτὸς μήτε τῆς ἡμέρης... ('lack of sleep, whether by night or

by day… ')[24] can be a predicting sign of imminent delirium (naturally, for him, delirium and sleep were unrelated). More remarkably, however, the author is acknowledging the existence of a good and a bad kind of sleep, thereby introducing its ambivalent status. Ultimately, three key concepts are enunciated in this passage: both excessive sleep and sleeplessness are detrimental, sleep is good during the night and insomnia is often associated with pain. In summary, like the author of *Prognosis* (and also the author of *On the sacred disease*), sleep can have positive or negative effects, but unlike them the process is completely alien to conditions where individuals are awake (that is, alert and hyperactive but disconnected, such as during hallucinations and delirium).[25]

The ambiguous status of sleep regarding health and disease also manifests in Aretaeus through its dual capacity of being a cure for certain conditions and at the same time a disease in its own right (as is the case with *lethargy*). Interestingly, he also took inspiration from the same passage of *Prognosis* to sustain the status of sleep as a cure for or prevention of delirium in *peripneumonia*:

ἢν δὲ ἄϋπνοι ἔωσι δι' ἡμέρης, ἠδὲ ἐγρηγορῶσι πάννυχοι, δέος μὴ ὁ ἄνθρωπος μανῇ, καὶ ποικίλων φαρμάκων ὑπνωτικῶν χρέος. *CA II.1. CMG (H).VI*: 120, 4–6.

If they are sleepless during the day and remain wakeful during the whole night, diverse sleep-inducing drugs are needed for fear of delirium.

Unlike Celsus, Aretaeus does maintain the Hippocratic conceptual relationship between sleep disturbances and delirium. As mentioned above, *phrenitis* is also a delirious condition that can be cured by sleep.[26]

In a similar manner, sleep is recommended as a treatment for *saturiasis*, a disease conceived as a permanent erection with delusion. The chapters tackling this particular condition offer an

---

[24] *Prog. CUF 10.3*: 27, 2–3.
[25] In terms of sleep patterns, this passage questions Nissin's (2016: 48) idea of a biphasic siesta culture among the Romans. If Celsus was actually discussing real social conventions, and not merely translating the Hippocratic author, his disapproval of sleep between the fourth hour and night-time speaks against an accepted culture of sleep during the *sexta hora*.
[26] ἢν γὰρ πάννυχοι μὲν ἐγρήσσωσι, μηδὲ δι' ἡμέρης εὕδωσι ('if they are wakeful the whole night, and cannot sleep in the day', *CA I.1. CMG (H)*: 94, 15–16). Of note is the similarity with the above-commented passage on *peripneumonia*.

Fuzzy edges, clear boundaries

interesting nuance about the author's conception of the peripheries of sleep. A subtle difference between its discussion in Aretaeus' book devoted to causes and signs and the one devoted to treatment reveals some interesting aspects about the nature of sleep. In the book on causes and signs ἴησις, ὕπνος βαθὺς καὶ μήκιστος. ψύξις γὰρ καὶ πάρεσις και νάρκη νεύρων, ὕπνος πολύς ('the cure is a deep and prolonged sleep. Indeed abundant sleep produces coldness, weakening and benumbing of the nerves').[27] In the book on treatment, on the other hand, Aretaeus suggests utilising abundant blood-letting, for οὐδὲ γὰρ ἄκαιρον νῦν λειποθυμίην ἐμποιέειν, ἔς τε νάρκην τῆς γνώμης ('it is not untimely to bring about fainting, in order to numb the gnômê')[28] (the disease was located in the nerves and the gnômê). In other words, a deep and prolonged sleep is equated to fainting, thereby blurring the boundaries between sleep and total loss of consciousness. It seems that for Aretaeus, the loss of consciousness that occurs with sleep is regarded as a treatment for diseases where there is hyperactive responsiveness, that is, the delirium characteristic of both *phrenitis* and *peripneumonia*, and the delusions of *saturiasis*.

The other side of the coin is sleep in and of itself – without being associated with delirium – regarded as the key symptom of a disease. Like Celsus and the author of the *Introduction*, Aretaeus construes *lethargy* as the perfect opposite of *phrenitis*. Accordingly, the treatment of *lethargy* is the exact antithesis of the former.

ληθαργικοῖσι κατάκλισις ἐν φωτὶ καὶ πρὸς αὐγήν· ζόφος γὰρ ἡ νοῦσος· ἠδὲ ἐν ἀλέῃ μᾶλλον· ψῦξις γὰρ ἔμφυτος ἡ αἰτίη. κοίτη εὐαφής, τοιχογραφίη, στρώματα ποικίλα, πάντα ὁκόσα περ ἐρεθιστικὰ ὄψιος, λαλιή, ψηλαφίη ξὺν πιέσι ποδῶν ... ἢν βαθὺ κῶμα ἴσχῃ, ἐμβόησις· νουθεσίη ὀργίλῃ· δεῖμα ἐφ'οἷσι δειμαίνει ... πάντα ἐς ἐγρήγορσιν ἐναντίως τοῖσι φρενιτικοῖσι. *CA I.2. CMG (H).V:* 98, 8–14.

For lethargic patients, lying in the light surrounded by brightness; darkness is actually the disease. Preferably warm, for innate cold is the cause. Soft bed, paintings on the walls, colourful bedclothes, whatever stimulates the sight, conversation, touching with compression on the feet ... If the patient falls into a deep stupor, shouts and angry reprimands [are needed] as well as threats about things that terrify them ... contrary to *phrenitis*, everything is aimed at waking them up.

---

[27] *SA II.11. CMG (H).II:* 34, 32; 35, 1–2.   [28] *CA II. 11. CMG (H).VI:* 142, 3–4.

The way in which the treatment is described – unfortunately the relevant chapter in the book of symptoms and causes is not extant – suggests that Aretaeus conceived two opposing affections of consciousness: one at the hyperactive end (*phrenitis*), in which perceptions were exacerbated and needed to be assuaged, and the other at the hypoactive end (*lethargy*), where the exact opposite stimuli (visual, auditory and tactile) were required (again, perceptions are a key part of his construction). In the middle of both is the grey area where hallucinations and delirium can be confused with nightmares. Accordingly, therapy through the spoken word is opposed; unlike the non-upsetting conversation recommended for *phrenetics*, *lethargy* warrants an aggressive and distressing approach.

Clearly, for both authors, at the centre of the definition of sleep is the kind of perceptions that are preserved and those that go unnoticed, which determine the model of disconnection conceived. They both distinguished a healthy and unhealthy type of sleep dependent on its amount (too much or too little were bad), and on the hour of the day in which it happened. Moreover, due to the post-Hellenistic redefinition of certain diseases, and the emergence of others, sleep became the cure for those with hyperactive impaired consciousness, mainly *phrenitis* (but also *saturiasis* in Aretaeus' account), and the main symptom of *lethargy*.

Some non-medical aspects of sleep

From a sociological point of view, beyond the seemingly well-established pattern of monophasic night-sleep in antiquity, the 'medicalisation' of excessive sleep and the 'pharmaceuticalisation'[29] of sleeplessness, the texts mention certain rituals, environments and artefacts, which suggest that in the real world the theoretical blurred limits of sleep were, perhaps, less vague.

Particularly, the overriding of certain conventions seems to indicate that relatives must have been clear regarding the status of a patient, whether he was sick or healthy, awake or asleep. Only through this assumption can one explain the normalisation of

---

[29] Williams (2008: 647).

'observed sleep during diseases'. Taylor points out that in a culture like ours, where sleep tends to be private, observed sleep reverts individuals to a powerless situation (like a baby or a patient).[30] Although we cannot automatically attribute the same connotations to the ancient descriptions, a passage by Galen (*Morb. Diff. II. K. VI*: 837, 5–10) that will be discussed later does suggest that sleeping was a quiet activity, with no external stimuli among healthy individuals. In other words, it would appear that infirmity operated also in antiquity as enough justification for intruding on an otherwise quiet and dark space. Similarly, aggressive therapies aimed at waking patients up from their *lethargy* broke the 'entitlement of the sleeper' (if such a thing ever existed in ancient societies).[31]

On the contrary, when sleep is construed as a remedy for hyperactive impaired consciousness (for example, *phrenitis*) or insomnia, all the conventions and rituals are enhanced, and intimate and quiet surroundings are encouraged or recreated. Aretaeus mentions some sleep-favouring environments in the treatment of *phrenitis*, when he relates that everyone finds delightful rest in their usual milieu (the sailor in his boat in the middle of the sea, the musician accompanied by music, the teacher amid the voices of his students).[32] Moreover, the sleeping arrangements to favour sleep in *phrenitis* (or wakefulness in *lethargy*) also reveal the practical artefacts available (soft or hard beds, colourful bedclothes, plain versus decorated walls, etc.). Although Celsus offers fewer details about these matters, he does refer to *suspensi lecti motus* ('hammocks, which [encourage sleep through their rocking] motion')[33] and *silanus iuxta cadens* ('the sound of falling water').[34]

All these details – which answer Taylor's questions How? Where? When? – show that, blurred as the boundaries between healthy and abnormal sleep might theoretically seem, once a diagnosis was reached (and therefore the ambiguity health/

---

[30] Taylor (1993: 466).

[31] According to Williams (2008: 642), in our society sleeping seems to be protected from disturbance in certain classes and ages.

[32] *CA I.1. CMG (H).V*: 94, 29–32; 95, 1–3.   [33] *Med. 3.18*: 15–18.

[34] *Med. 3.18*: 15. Perhaps he is referring to the *impluvium* in the traditional Roman *domus*? In any case, Nissin (2016: 32–5) did not make any allusion to it in her in-depth analysis of sleeping spaces within Roman houses.

disease vanished), completely opposing practical approaches were put into place (the same could be said regarding the ambiguity between wakefulness and sleep). As a result, it is reasonable to speculate that in the face of actual cases all the ambiguities needed to be resolved, and patients ended up being classified as either having healthy or disturbed sleep, and as either suffering from vivid dreams or wakeful hallucinations. Accordingly, the corresponding measures were put into place (for example, a quiet, comfortable environment, soft mattresses, plain walls and pleasant talk for favouring sleep versus shouts, prodding, hard mattresses and colourful bedding to prevent it).

Levels of consciousness

In accordance with his conception of sleep as an all-or-nothing phenomenon, there is only one passage in which Celsus seems to acknowledge different depths, and relates deep and disturbed sleep to more severe diseases. When discussing predictor signs of illness he mentions:

si gravior somnus pressit, si tumultuosa somnia fuerunt, si saepius expergiscitur aliquis quam adsuevit, deinde iterum soporatur... *Med.* 2.2: 2.

if heavier sleep oppresses, if there are unsettling dreams, if somebody wakes up more often than usual and then becomes drowsy again...

In most other cases, Celsus seems to have regarded sleep and wakefulness as mutually exclusive phenomena, and accordingly, we can find in his work no further attempts at distinguishing different levels of drowsiness. Moreover, in the discussion on *lethargy*, the lack of interest in the depth of sleep becomes particularly evident. He utilises no adverbs, comparative adjectives or any other linguistic resource to nuance different degrees or intensities. It seems as though for Celsus the patient can be either asleep or awake but there are no intermediate states.[35]

---

[35] Mudry (2006c: 138–9) has studied how Celsus distinguishes between mortal and severe diseases, and among the latter, how he refers to the different degrees of severity through adverbs and comparative degrees of adjectives. Such rhetorical devices are not used to talk about sleep.

On the contrary, Aretaeus' endeavours to define different levels of consciousness are particularly evident in his characterisation of *peripneumonia*:

Ἢν δὲ ἐπὶ τὸ θανατῶδες ἐπιδιδοῖ, ἀγρυπνίη, ὕπνοι σμικροί, νωθροί, κωματώδεες, φαντασίαι ἀξύνετοι· παράληροι τὴν γνώμην ἐκστατικοὶ οὐ μάλα. *SA II.1. CMG (H).II*: 16, 8–10.

If [the disease] becomes terminal, there is restlessness, interrupted sleep, sluggishness, stupor, unintelligible visions. Sufferers are deluded in their *gnômê*, although not extremely deranged.

The accumulation of nouns, qualifiers and adverbs suggests that Aretaeus is trying to describe different and apparently increasing levels of drowsiness. Considering that the condition seems to be reaching a deadly (*thanatôdes*) stage one could even suggest a correlation between severity of the disease and degree of disconnection, although this is less explicit than in the Hippocratic collection. Be that as it may, in clear agreement with the Hippocratic doctors, the author is describing discrete stages or levels of consciousness. Moreover, apart from the patient becoming progressively less reactive, he seems to be suffering – as part of the same phenomenon – *phantasiai axunetoi* and *paralêroi tên gnômên*, thereby, again, blurring the boundaries between delirium, wakeful hallucinations and visions in dreams.

Terminology and HOFs

As in the HC, the use of terminology among these authors is also revealing of their ideas about the workings of the mind. We have been seeing in the analysis of both hallucinations and sleep how perceptions acquired increasing relevance among post-Hellenistic authors (possibly connected to new insights into the functioning of the nervous system developed during the Hellenistic period).

Naturally, due to their abridged nature, HOFs are scarcely elaborated in the *Introduction* and the *Medical definitions*. Nevertheless, their compilers did associate a disturbed *dianoia* with descriptions of *phrenitis* and *mania*.[36] In the cases of Celsus and Aretaeus, there seems to be more reflection on the topic.

Although Celsus' understanding of the mind and the soul are radically different from the ideas that emerged from the Hippocratic authors, it is precisely in the passages that show strong Hippocratic influence that his conceptions appear more clearly. Indeed, his use of partial synonymy and his coinage of phrasal terms, which follow (from a formal point of view) rather closely some Hippocratic models, reveal his underlying (un-Hippocratic) ideas on these matters. Similarly, in Aretaeus' work we can see a use of language that reminds us of the HC; however, such similarities are only restricted to the formal aspects.

Persistent use of partial synonymy

A common practice among scholars has been to find correspondences between *On medicine* and some Hippocratic texts. By using this technique, Stok and Pigeaud have convincingly argued that the term *delirium* in Celsus is sometimes used as an equivalent of *paraphrosunê* and sometimes of *parakopê*.[37] I propose to reverse the method; in other words, to apply it in the opposite manner, in order to see which other words in Celsus' text are used to talk about delirium (my emphasis):

si quid etiam abscessit, et antequam suppuraret manente adhuc febre subsedit, periculum adfert primum **furoris**, deinde interitus. auris quoque dolor

---

[36] As noted, *phrenitis* was defined as: ἔκστασις διανοίας μετὰ παρακοπῆς σφοδρᾶς (*Int. CUF 13.9:* 51, 4–5) and παρακοπὴ διανοίας . . . καὶ διανοίας ἔκστασις (*Def. Med. 234. K. XIX:* 412, 17–18), whereas *mania* was defined as: περὶ τὴν διάνοιαν ἐκστάσεως· (*Int. CUF 13.24:* 57, 6–7) and ἔκστασις τῆς διανοίας (*Def. Med. 246. K.XIX:* 416, 8).

[37] Pigeaud (1994: 267), and Stok (1996: 2336) juxtaposed *On medicine* with *Aphorisms* (my emphasis):

neque is servari potest . . . *qui febre aeque non quiescent simul et **delirio** et spirandi difficultate vexatur* (*Med. 2.6:* 7).

ὅκου ἐν πυρετῷ μὴ διαλείποντι δύσπνοια γίνεται καὶ **παραφροσύνη**, θανάσιμον (*Aph. LCL IV.50:* 148).

aestiva quartana fere brevis est, cui calor et tremor est, saluti *delirium* est (*Med. 2.8:* 16).

ὁκόσοισιν ἂν ἐν τοῖσι καύσοισι τρόμοι γένωνται, **παρακοπὴ** λύει (*Aph. LCL VI.26:* 184).

acutus cum febre continua vehementique saepe **mentem turbat** ... suffusae quoque sanguine mulieris mammae **furorem** venturum esse testantur. *Med. 2.7: 26–7.*

Moreover, if an abscess appears, and before it suppurates it [the abscess] starts decreasing while the fever persists, it carries the risk first of delirium (*furoris*), then of death. Also, acute earache with continuously elevated fever often disturbs the *mens* (*mentem turbat*) ... Women's breasts, when flooded with blood, also attest to the fact that delirium (*furorem*) is about to occur.

This extract belongs to the second book within the dietetics section, where Celsus discusses generalities about diseases. In this particular passage he is addressing bad prognostic signs specific to certain ailments. Stok has shown how Celsus condensed within it three different fragments from the Hippocratic corpus.[38] The first appearance of *furor* corresponds to *paraphronêsê* in *Prognosis 18.6*, the second one to *maniên* in *Aphorisms V.40*. *Mentem turbat*, finally, is Celsus' equivalent of *paraphronêsai* as it appears in *Prognosis 22.1*. The synonymy between *furor* and *mentem turbare*, therefore, is not only clear through comparison with their Greek sources, but also by the context in which they appear, for the repetition of the adverb *quoque* also suggests that they have similar meanings. Furthermore, Celsus recaps later in the pharmacological section of his work a fragment of this passage and paraphrases it:

aurium inflammationes doloresque interdum etiam ad **dementiam** mortemque praecipitant *Med. 6.7:* 1A.

pain and inflammation of the ears often trigger delirium (dementiam) and death.

In this way, *dementia* also seems to correspond to *paraphronêsai* in *Prognosis 22.1*, thereby becoming yet another partial synonym

---

[38] Stok (1996: 1335–6). Below are the three passages (my emphasis):
1. ἢν δὲ ἀφανίζωνται ... αἱ ἀποστάσιες, τοῦ πτυέλου μὴ ἐκχωρέοντος τοῦ τε πυρετοῦ ἔχοντος, δεινόν· κίνδυνος γαρ, μὴ **παραφρονήσῃ** καὶ ἀποθάνῃ ὁ ἄνθρωπος (*Prog. CUF 18.6:* 53, 10–12; 54, 1–2).
2. γυναιξὶν ὁκόσῃσιν ἐς τοὺς τιτθοὺς αἷμα συστρέφεται, **μανίην** σημαίνει (*Aph. LCL V.40:* 168).
3. ὠτὸς δὲ ὀδύνη ὀξεῖη ξὺν πυρετῷ συνεχεῖ τε καὶ ἰσχυρῷ δεινόν· **παραφρονῆσαι** γὰρ κίνδυνος τὸν ἄνθρωπον καὶ ἀπολέσθαι (*Prog. CUF 22.1:* 63, 1–3).

of *furor* as well as *turbare mentem* (and also of *delirium* if we take into account Stok and Pigeaud's above-mentioned deductions). This use of partial synonymy suggests that – much like the Hippocratic doctors (albeit with a smaller number of terms) – Celsus also perceived the very nature of delirium as changing and variable. Like them, and as with present usage, these partial synonyms express subtle nuances – often difficult to define – within a broader continuum of wakeful impaired consciousness.[39]

Another important aspect that these correspondences reveal is the intervention of the *mens* in wakeful impaired consciousness, both in the compound *dementiam* (with the negative prefix *de-*) and in the phrasal term *turbare mentem*. We shall see below that this concept, along with *animus* (and less frequently *consilium*) – which Celsus used interchangeably in his discussion on *insania* (*Med. 3.18*: 19–21) – are comprised of several HOFs and play an important role in his idea of consciousness.

In the case of Aretaeus, the sleep and delirium terminology also reflects his ideas about the mind, and partial synonymy is still present, even if the vocabulary has also been quantitatively reduced (that is, he utilises fewer words than the HC to discuss impaired consciousness). In this sense, I disagree with Pigeaud and Murphy, who argue that *mainomai* only refers to the delusions that characterise *mania*.[40] On the contrary, in some passages discussed above *mainomai* appears in the discussion on *phrenitis*, where it is semantically equivalent to *paraphorê*,[41] and in the distinction between substance-induced delirium and *mania*, where *ekmainomai* and *paraphorê* are again used interchangeably.[42]

There are, however, certain nuances. The concept of *lêrêsis*, which was also a partial synonym of all these terms in the HC, has now become an independent entity: it refers to a disease in its own right (which we would now associate with dementia of the elderly).[43]

[39] I do not think that the alternation between terms is necessarily a case of *variatio sermonis*, which is, otherwise, a recurring feature of Celsus' style (Mudry 1994: 137).
[40] Pigeaud (1987: 84), Murphy (2013: 19).   [41] *CA 1. CMG (H).V*: 91, 16–17; 92, 1–2.
[42] *SD I.6. CMG (H).III*: 41, 15–17.   [43] *SD I.6. CMG (H).III*: 41, 19.

Phrasal terms, HOFs and the organisation of the mind

The use of phrasal terms is particularly revealing of Celsus' theoretical framework, especially because, in *On medicine*, such periphrastic constructions are less lexicalised than in the Hippocratic corpus.[44] Unlike the Greek technical vocabulary that was better developed and had become estranged from etymology, Celsus explicitly complained about the scarcity of Latin terminology, which led him to make careful choices in his vocabulary while trying to avoid polysemy.[45] As a result, when he refers to delirium with *turbare mentem* (*Med. 2.7*: 27) and *dementia* (*Med. 6.7*: 1A), the disturbance that he envisaged actually did affect what he understood to be the *mens*. Its compromise is expressed through other phrasal terms. Examples abound in descriptions of diseases with impaired consciousness:[46] in *insania* the *mens labat* ('the *mens* declines', *Med. 3.19*: 1); in *apoplêxia* – which is a case of hypoactive impaired consciousness – the *mens stupet* ('the *mens* is stunned', *Med. 3.26*); in hot weather the *mens hebetat* ('the *mens* is weakened', *Med. 2.1*: 11); and in *kephalaian* there is *alienatio mentis* ('aberration of the *mens*', *Med. 4.2*: 2). Some of these phrasal terms even have a direct correlation with the Hippocratic corpus. For instance a passage of *On medicine* where *mens labat*[47] matches a Hippocratic one where *gnômê noseei*,[48] thereby suggesting a correspondence between *mens* and *gnômê*.

The relevance of the *mens* for normal cognitive functioning is also emphasised in situations where consciousness is preserved (that is, in the 'vocabulary of lucidity'). Thus it is possible that after *insania*, *mens redit* ('the *mens* returns', *Med. 3.18*: 23); in *cardiacum* the body is affected but the *mens constat* ('the *mens* remains firm', *Med. 3.19*: 1); in cold weather *mens erectior est* ('the *mens* is more elevated', *Med. 2.1*: 11); and a good sign after a wound is when *mens consistit* ('the *mens* resists', *Med. 5.26*:

---

[44] Langslow (1994: 305).   [45] Langslow (1994: 300).
[46] Gourevitch (1991: 564) has remarked that *delirium* and *desipere* are similar cases.
[47] ... *quibus causa doloris neque sensus eius est, his **mens labat*** ('... for those who, having a cause for pain, do not feel it', my emphasis) (*Med. 2.7*: 21).
[48] ὁκόσοι, πονέοντές τι τοῦ σώματος, τὰ πολλὰ τῶν πόνων μὴ αἰσθάνονται, τούτοισιν ἡ γνώμη νοσεῖ (*Aph. LCL II.6*: 110, 1–2).

26A). Throughout all these examples, *mens* seems to refer to different intellectual capacities, apart from 'la faculté de penser'.[49]

Furthermore, as stated in the discussion on *insania*, *animus* and *mens* are used interchangeably. Not surprisingly, there are also phrasal terms where the noun head is *animus*. Thus, fever-associated delirium is expressed as *animus laborat* ('the *animus* suffers', *Med. 3.5*: 11); in *phthisis* it is advisable to avoid anything that can *sollicitare animum* ('disturb the *animus*', *Med. 3.22*: 9). Finally, successful treatments in *phrenesis* – in which *mens* ... *[vanibus] imaginibus addicta est* ('the *mens* has succumbed to empty visions')[50]– contribute *ad quietem animi* ('to the repose of the *animus*', *Med. 3.18*: 5), and some *phrenitic* patients that are offered a treatment through the spoken word begin to *convertere animum* ('change their *animus*', *Med. 3.18*: 11).

When trying to delimit the scope of these terms, it becomes evident that sense-perception was often included within the notion of *mens* (a few excerpts, as well as the *vanas imagines* of *phrenesis*, testify to this).[51] Other examples suggest that *mens* was involved in the faculty of rational thought. This is particularly evident in the distinction made between the two subspecies of the third kind of *insania*: in the first one individuals perceive *imagines* even though their *mens* is intact, and therefore they can reason (the examples given are Orestes' and Ajax's delusion).[52] In the other subtype, where *mens* is used interchangeably with *animus* and *consilium*, their derangement makes the patient *perperam aliquid dixit aut fecit* ('speak or act wrongly'),[53] which can point towards an alteration in judgement, speech or both.[54]

In summary, *mens* is one among few other abstract terms (such as *animus*) used by Celsus to discuss HOFs or ideas akin to what we would nowadays include within the sphere of cognition and associate

---

[49] Gourevitch (1991: 565).   [50] *Med. 3.18*: 3.

[51] Based on the correspondences *gnômê–mens* and *marmarugai–imagines*, Pigeaud (1994: 271–3) posited that madness was only a matter of perception, and that Celsus was referring to contemporary philosophical debates about the reality of such perceptions.

[52] I disagree with Harris (2013a: 304) that *imagines* exclusively refers to visual hallucinations. From what we know about Ajax and Orestes, such apparitions were also auditory.

[53] *Med. 3.18*: 21.

[54] As discussed above, the association between speech disturbances and *mens* can also be illustrated by the example of the treatment for gangrene (*Med. 5.26*: 14E).

with consciousness. Although perceptions do play a privileged role in the genesis of *phrenesis*, on the more theoretical level, *mens* seems to subsume – much like the Hippocratic notions of *gnômê*, *nous*, *phronêsis*, etc. – different capacities in different contexts, amongst which perceptions do not have a higher hierarchy than judgement, reasoning or speech.[55]

Aretaeus' understanding of the mind, on the other hand, is strongly influenced by the opposition of *gnômê* and *aisthêsis*. This organisation of mental capacities emerges quite clearly from his distinction between delirium and mental illness. The contrast between *phrenitis* and *mania/melancholia*, which he strongly emphasised, suggests a dichotomous division of HOFs. He opposed the affection of the *aisthêsis* (located in the head, which triggered the hallucinations that characterised *phrenitis*) to a compromise of the *gnômê* (that caused impaired emotions, behaviours and thinking, by affecting the heart). In this manner he separated two main areas of cognitive functioning, thereby also avoiding taking a clear side in the encephalocentric versus cardiocentric debate: faithful to his lax eclecticism, he adhered to both. Indeed, particularly in discussions concerning what we now define as mental disease, *gnômê* is presented in opposition to *aisthêsis* as its complementary counterpart, as though Aretaeus was suggesting a dichotomous idea of the mind comprised of *aisthêsis* and *gnômê*.[56] This way of fragmenting the HOFs makes Aretaeus' understanding more compatible with some Hellenistic conceptions about the nervous system.[57] However, as I mentioned before, there are also examples of syncretism that challenge the previous view (which should not surprise us considering his lax eclecticism).

Such is the passage where Aretaeus describes the above-normal perceptions that occur due to extreme dryness in *kausôn* ('the

---

[55] Although up until this point in the analysis Celsus' idea of *mens/animus* might not seem to contradict most Hippocratic authors, I shall argue in Part III that his conception of mind (*animus/mens*) – particularly in opposition to *anima* – has a strong Epicurean influence, which distances him from them.

[56] If we were to think of this scheme in Stoic terms, Aretaeus would be removing the sense-perception capacity from the comprehensive Stoic *hêgemonikon*, located in the heart (where he placed *mania-melancholia*), and sending it to the head and the nerves (namely, the primary *locus affectus* in *phrenitis*).

[57] Annas (1992: 64–89).

aisthêsis is absolutely pure, the *dianoia* subtle and the *gnômê* prophetic', *SA II. CMG (H).II*: 24, 2–3). According to this description, he divided the cognitive functions into three (instead of two): *aisthêsis*, *dianoia* and *gnômê*. This tripartition also appears in the chapter that addresses epilepsy: δυσμαθέες νωθείη γνώμης τε καὶ αἰσθήσιος ... ὑποτείνεται δέ κοτε καὶ τὴν διάνοιαν ἡ νοῦσος, ὡς τὰ πάντα μωραίνειν ('they are slow at learning, with sluggishness in their *gnômê* and their *aisthêsis* ... sometimes the disease strains the *dianoia* so that they become completely foolish').[58] Although expanded – as compared to the binary fragmentation that characterised the contrast *phrenitis–mania/melancholia* – the picture would still not be completely incompatible with the previous dichotomous opposition between *aisthêsis* and *gnômê*. The mind, in this case, would be divided into perceptions or *aisthêsis*, which are affected by diseases such as *phrenitis*; *gnômê*, which controls behaviours and emotions and is impaired in *mania–melancholia*; and finally, *dianoia*, which seems to refer to reason or the capacity to think.

However, on other occasions new components are mentioned. In the distinction between *mania* and *lêrêsis* of the elderly, the latter affects *aisthêsis*, *gnômê* and *nous*: λήρησις αἰσθήσιος γάρ ἐστι νάρκη, καὶ γνώμης νάρκωσις ἡδὲ τοῦ νοῦ ὑπὸ ψύξιος ('[it] is numbness of *aisthêsis* and benumbing of both the *gnômê* and the *nous* due to cold'),[59] whereas in the *prooemium* to the books on chronic illnesses Aretaeus only separates *aisthêsis* and *psuchê*: ἀλλ᾽ ἐς πολλὰ τὴν αἰσθησίην ἐκτρέπει, ἀλλὰ καὶ τὴν ψυχὴν ἐκμαίνει ('not only do [bad mixtures of the body] often alter perceptions, but they delude (*ekmainei*) the *psuchê* as well').[60] Moreover, in the discussion on *phrenitis*, apart from the *aisthêsis* that I have already mentioned, there are allusions to the *thumos* and the *phrên*. The *thumos* is μειλίγματα γὰρ θυμοῦ σιτία ('Food is melody for the *thumos*')[61] or ἄριστος δὲ μειλίξαι θυμὸν ἐν παραφορῇ ([wine] 'best sets the *thumos* to music during delirium (*paraphorê*)'), that is, wine and food appease the spirit.[62] The *phrên*, on the other hand,

---

[58] *SD I.4. CMG (H).III*: 39, 4–5, 8–9.   [59] *SD I.6. CMG (H).III*: 41, 19–20.
[60] *SD I.1. CMG (H).III*: 36, 16–17.
[61] *CA I.1. CMG (H).V*: 92, 9.
[62] *CA I.1. CMG (H).V*: 97, 28).

could be regarded as an example of *sumphorêsis*: it refers in one passage to an HOF affected by vinous fruits,[63] and it designates the diaphragm in another.[64]

It could be argued, therefore, that despite a clear isolation of the *aisthêsis* as an independent key component of consciousness (and consciousness-affecting diseases), there is – as among the Hippocratic doctors – vagueness, overlapping and inconsistencies in Aretaeus' descriptions of the other mental capacities (albeit with a reduced terminology, for *phronêsis* and *sunesis* do not appear in his lexicon).

Despite all these nuances, whenever Aretaeus wants to convey the idea of delirium or confusion in contexts where specific capacities are less relevant, that is, when he does not need to differentiate impaired consciousness from other specific cognitive compromises, he uses phrasal terms where *gnômê* is the nominal head. In *peripneumonia* there is *gnômês aporiê* ('puzzled *gnômê*', *SA II.1. CMG (H).II*: 16, 7); during acute affections of the liver the *gnômê ou karta paraphoros* ('the *gnômê* is not extremely delirious', *SA II.6. CMG (H).II*: 27, 27–8); in an acute disease of the hollow vein, patients are *tên gnômên ou paraphoroi* ('not delirious in their *gnômê*, *SA II.8. CMG (H).II*: 29, 21); in suppurating diseases they are *tên gnômên paralêroi* ('delirious in their *gnômê*', *SD I.9. CMG (H).III*: 50, 12). On the contrary, in whiter jaundices patients become *gnômê de phaidroteroi* ('brighter in their *gnômê*', *SD I.15. CMG (H).III*: 59, 12).

It seems that *gnômê* is used in two different ways: as a general term to convey the idea of impaired consciousness, when no further nuances are needed, and as a more specific term to distinguish mental illness or delusion (which affect the *gnômê*) from impaired consciousness due to altered perceptions (in which *gnômê* is opposed to *aisthêsis*).

In summary, the analysis of HOFs reinforces what has already been said when analysing hallucinations and sleep. Aretaeus'

---

[63] ὀπώρης οἰνώδεος ... κεφαλῆς γὰρ καὶ φρενῶν ἄψιν ποιέει ('vinous fruits ... affect the head and the *phrênes*', *CA I.1. CMG (H).V*: 93, 24). Note that this phrasal term is also used by the author of the Hippocratic treatise *On diseases of women I* (*Mul. I. LCL 63*: 134, 1) to talk about delirium.

[64] θυμὸν τε γὰρ πρηΰνονται μαλθάξει φρενῶν ('fomentations are to be applied to the *phrên* in order to soften the *thumos*', *CA I.1. CMG (H).V*: 97, 28).

stress on disturbed perceptions as a key feature to explain diseases where consciousness was compromised is paralleled by the key role of *aisthêsis* as an independent capacity in the way he fragments the HOFs. When comparing his stance to Celsus', we can still see the difference in emphasis that was highlighted in relation to the clinical presentation. Celsus only considered altered perceptions to be a key finding when addressing the symptoms, but they did not have a privileged status in his theoretical constructs such as *mens* or *animus*. In them, perceptions were just one component among others. Aretaeus, on the other hand, not only stressed the relevance of hallucinations in his clinical characterisation of the diseases, but also conceived *aisthêsis* as an individual HOF with the same hierarchy as, for instance, *gnômê*.

CHAPTER 10

SLEEP IN GALEN

In line with his strict distinction between processes according or contrary to nature, in Galen's comprehensive system there is less room for ambiguities: health and disease are clearly separated, and disease is characterised by a *locus affectus*, a specific type of imbalance, and a quantitative degree of imbalance.

Boundaries between health and disease: natural versus non-natural sleep

Naturally, this author recognised healthy sleep and a non-healthy state, *kôma*, which could be wakeful or drowsy. The normal process is described in *On the distinction of diseases*:

... ἐπεὶ καὶ κοιμώμενοι, καὶ ἄλλως ἐν σκότῳ καὶ ἡσυχίᾳ διάγοντες, ἢ κατακείμενοι πολλάκις οὔτε τι μέρος κινοῦμεν, οὔθ᾽ ὅλως αἰσθανόμεθα τῶν ἔξωθεν οὐδενός, οὐδὲν μὴν ἧττον ὑγιαίνομεν. *Morb. Diff. II. K.VI*: 837, 5–10.

... when we sleep and spend time in the darkness, quietly lying, often without moving any part, and perceiving absolutely nothing from outside, we are not less healthy.

This is the passage mentioned above where sleep is described as a quiet activity: in the dark, without external stimuli (which would suggest that observed sleep was an unusual situation). On a more physiological note, disconnection from the environment (*tôn exôthen*) is a crucial feature of sleep. Apart from perceptions – which had appeared in Aretaeus – Galen highlights the lack of movement. Considering that both are capacities of the *psuchê* in Galen's theoretical model, it is not surprising that the unhealthy kind of sleep will be considered together with the conditions that affect the ruling part of the soul (located in the brain):

... καὶ πρὸς τούτοις ἔτι δύο ἐξαίρετα, τὸ μὲν ἀγρυπνία, τὸ δὲ κῶμα ... ἐφεξῆς δ᾽ ἂν εἴη τὰς τῶν ἡγεμονικῶν ἐνεργειῶν βλάβας διελθεῖν ... ἔστι δὲ καὶ ταύτης ... ὃ δὲ κάρος καὶ κατάληψις . . . τὸ δὲ οἷον ἐλλιπὴς καὶ ἄτονος [κίνησις], ὡς ἐν κώμασί τε καὶ ληθάργοις. . . *Symp. Diff. CMG 3.6*: 220, 23; 221, 1. *K.VII*: 58; *3.9*: 224, 9–10. *K. VII*: 60.

. . . apart from these [damages common to all perceptual activities], there are also two special ones: sleeplessness and *kôma* . . . Subsequently, the damages to the *hêgemonikon* [itself] should be discussed . . . Amongst [those that affect imagination] are . . . torpor (*karos*) and *catalepsy* . . . [and] something akin to a defective [movement] lacking tone, as in *kômas* and *lethargies*. . .

In a nutshell, non-natural sleep occurs when the *psuchê* is either affected in the *aisthêtikon* or the *phantastikon* (which in turn belongs to the *hêgemonikon*). Hence, the *locus affectus* is clear, and with it, the site to which the treatment should be applied:

καὶ μὲν δὴ κἀπὶ τῶν ληθαργικῶν οὐδείς ἐστιν ὃς οὐ προσφέρει τῇ κεφαλῇ τὰ βοηθήματα· καὶ τοῦτο γὰρ τὸ πάθος . . . γίνεται δ᾽ ἐγκεφάλου πάσχοντος, ἐν ᾧ τῆς ψύχης ἐστι τὸ ἡγεμονικόν. *MM XIII.21. LCL III*: 400, 26–7; 402,1–2. *K.X*: 929.

neither is there anybody who would not apply the treatment to the head in *lethargic* patients, for this affection also . . . occurs when the brain, where the *hêgemonikon* of the *psuchê* lies, suffers.

Sleep and wakefulness as a continuum

The consequence of the above-mentioned disturbances is designated as *kôma* or *kataphora*, namely, impaired consciousness:

. . . δύο εἰσὶν εἴδη καταφορᾶς . . . commune enim ambabus est, quia elevare non possunt oculos, sed mox gravantur et dormire volunt, proprium autem alterius, quia hii quidem dormiunt mox et profunde et diu hii vero vigiles versute sunt, alia super aliam fantasiam adveniente et mentem movente et somnum incidente . . . sive igitur somnolenta sive vigil fuerit catafora, vocare coma est consuetudo ei, et nequaquam sibi invicem repugnant . . ., quandoque quidem in vigiliis parvis invenietur coma quandoque autem in somno. etenim et catafora quandoque quidem somnolenta est, quandoque autem vigil; quare non habes dicere de catafora patientibus, quod vigilant vel non.[1] *Hipp. Com. CMG II*: 187, 12–18; 29–33; 188, 1–2. *K.VII*: 653–4.

---

[1] The change from Greek into Latin follows the edition by Mewaldt, Diels and Heeg in the *CMG V: 9.2*. Melwadt explains (*Praefatio XIV–XV*) that the only extant version of the text was the *Codex Laurentianus* 74,3 from the twelfth century, which had a large *lacuna*. In order to solve it they used a Latin translation from the fourteenth century by Nicolao de Regio de Calabria (*Codex Parisinus* 6865) which, unlike Kuhn's edition, filled the *lacuna* with a reverse translation from Latin back into Greek. The passage transcribed is found exactly at the beginning of this *lacuna*, hence most of the text is in Latin.

Sleep and wakefulness as a continuum

... drowsiness (*kataphora*) presents in two forms ... common to both [of them] is the fact that [patients] cannot open their eyes but are soon weighed down and wish to sleep; but specific to one [form] is the fact that the former [sufferers from *kôma*] fall asleep quickly and deeply during the day, while the latter [sufferers from *kataphora*] are actually deceitfully awake, for dreamy apparitions come to their mind (*mens*) and move it, thereby interrupting their sleep ... Regardless of whether the drowsiness (*kataphora*) is somnolent or wakeful we customarily call it *kôma*, and by no means do they [the two forms] oppose each other ... *kôma* is sometimes found in short wakeful periods, and sometimes in sleep. Indeed, also drowsiness (*kataphora*) is sometimes somnolent and sometimes wakeful, wherefore you should not say whether patients who suffer drowsiness are awake or not.

The transition between abnormal sleep and wakefulness is so blurred that in conditions with impaired consciousness one cannot really tell one from the other. As a matter of fact, Galen is suggesting that it makes no sense trying to distinguish between them. In contemporary terms we would construe the concept as a single condition (*kataphora*, *kôma*, impaired consciousness) with various manifestations (drowsiness, hallucinations, confusion). Furthermore, such a view actually implies that somnolent and wakeful impaired consciousness are two presentations of a similar phenomenon. This stance is not only in utter contradiction to Celsus, who conceived sleep as an all-or-nothing phenomenon (where patients could only be either awake or asleep), but it also challenges the Hippocratic authors and Aretaeus. Indeed, although all of them did admit some grey areas with fuzzy edges between wakefulness and sleep, they nonetheless attempted to associate such conditions either with one or the other (as discussed within the sociological commentary, the specific treatment for each category required that kind of clarity in the classification).[2]

The blurred boundaries, however, are not limited to the distinction between delirium and sleep. A passage where Galen contrasted certain diseases of the *hêgemonikon* with *sunkopê* illuminates the way in which he understood the relationship between the three prototypes of impaired consciousness:

οὕτω γοῦν ἐπιληψίαι τε διὰ τὸν ἄτονον στόμαχον ἐνίοις ἐπιγίνονται, καὶ κάροι, καὶ κώματα, καὶ καταλήψεις, παραφροσύναι τε καὶ μελαγχολίαι, τῆς κατὰ τὸν ἐγκέφαλόν τε καὶ τὰ νεῦρα συμπαθούσης ἀρχῆς. αἱ δὲ ὀνομαζόμεναι καρδιακαὶ

---

[2] *On internal diseases* (*LCL 48*) offers a good example, where the author is also explicitly trying to separate hallucinations from nightmares.

συγκοπαὶ τῆς κατὰ τὴν καρδίαν τε καὶ τὰς ἀρτηρίας ἀρχῆς συμπαθούσης ἐπιγίγνονται. *Caus. Symp. I.7. K.VII*: 137, 5–11.

In this way, epilepsy falls upon some due to a weak stomach, as do torpors (*karoi*), *kômas*, catalepsies (*katalêpseis*), deliria (*paraphrosunai*) and bouts of *melancholia*, providing there is *sympathy* towards the principle (*archê*) located in the brain and the nerves. The so-called cardiac *sunkopai* supervene as long as the *sympathy* occurs towards the principle (*archê*) located in the heart and the arteries.

First of all, the fact that Galen needed to contrast conditions with impaired *hêgemonikon* and *phantastikon* – such as *epilepsy, torpor, kôma, catalepsy* and delirium – with *cardiacum* (total loss of consciousness) suggests that he perceived them to be easily confused conditions.[3] In terms of their specific links, the three prototypes of impaired consciousness may well originate in the stomach, but they all ultimately affect a part of his tripartite soul: the *psuchê*.[4] The difference is that whereas the latter has sympathy towards the *archê* in the heart (spirited *psuchê*), all the others have it towards the brain (rational *psuchê*). The kind of disease that develops depends on where specifically the *sympathy* goes.

In other words, the problem begins in the stomach, but it is the second stopover that will determine the kind of affection: if it is the rational soul, it will trigger diseases of the *hêgemonikon* (with drowsy or hyperactive impaired consciousness), whereas if the spirited soul receives the *sympathy*, it will trigger a *sunkopê* (total loss of consciousness). The above shows that although the *psuchê* was affected in all the situations that we nowadays consider as impaired consciousness, there were nuances. As we shall see in Part III of this book, Galen consistently attributed delirium and sleep to the *hêgemonikon*, whereas fainting was sometimes related to a different part of his tripartite Platonic soul. When the emphasis was put on the loss of movement and perceptions that fainting

---

[3] Note Galen's preference for describing specific deficiencies attributable to determined *loci affecti* that he could target with the treatment: he considered that epilepsy was a spasm combined with cessation of the functions of the *hêgemonikon*, whereas *karos* and *katalepseis* were a paralysis of the *phantastikon*, both anatomically located in the brain.

[4] In the chapters on delirium I have discussed why I consider *melancholia* to be a form of mental illness and not impaired consciousness. The fact that in this passage Galen includes it among the others can be explained in terms of his system: regardless of the actual symptoms, it was a cold and moist *duskrasia* in the brain, and as such it could be triggered by *sympathy* from the stomach.

causes, the affection of the *hêgemonikon* in the brain was emphasised. When, on the other hand the mechanism of swoons (the loss of blood) was under discussion, the attention was diverted towards the spirited soul in the heart, which carries the innate heat.

Levels of consciousness

For certain, Galen offers explicit speculation on the gradable physiology of both healthy and pathological sleep. As far as the former is concerned,

... κατὰ τοὺς ὕπνους ἤτοι παντάπασιν ἀργοῦσιν αἱ αἰσθήσεις, ἢ ἀμυδρῶς ἐνεργοῦσιν. εὔλογον οὖν ὀλίγην τινα ἐπιρρεῖν τηνικαῦτα δύναμιν ἀπὸ τῆς ἀρχῆς τοῖς κατὰ μέρος. καὶ τό γε βαθέως τε καὶ μὴ βαθέως κοιμᾶσθαι ... ἐν τῷ ποσῷ τῆς ἐπιρροῆς ἐστι. τοσούτῳ γὰρ μεῖον ἐπιρρεῖν εἰκός ἐστιν, ὅσῳπερ ἂν ὁ ὕπνος ᾖ βαθύτερος. *Caus. Symp. I.7. K.VII:* 140, 4–10.

... during sleep, perceptions are either completely inactive, or they operate weakly. Hence, it is reasonable that in such circumstances there is little capacity flowing from the controlling centre towards them [the perception organs]. To fall asleep deeply and non-deeply depends on the amount of the flow: the lesser the flow, the deeper the sleep.

Galen explicitly conceives different levels of disconnection that manifest in progressive depths of sleep, and they depend on the quantity of perception capacity flowing from the *archê* (in the brain) towards the senses.

Concerning the abnormal kind of sleep, I have already pointed out that in Galen's system, the antithetic character of the qualities (cold–hot, dry–moist) enables a rational explanation for opposite symptoms (such as insomnia–drowsiness). We should now add that the gradual nature of such qualities allows – and even encourages – reflection upon their intensity. For certain, qualities admit degrees, which makes it relatively easy for a doctor to correlate levels of heat, coldness, dryness or moistness to a corresponding severity of the compromise:

ὥσπερ οὖν ὕπνος καὶ ἀγρυπνία μᾶλλον τοῦ μετρίου γίνεται, τὸ μὲν δι᾽ ὑγρότητα, τὸ δὲ διὰ ξηρότητα κράσεως, οὕτως ἐν αὐτοῖς τούτοις τὸ μᾶλλόν τε καὶ ἧττον ἐν ἀγρυπνίαις τε καὶ ὕπνοις ἔπεται τῷ μᾶλλον καὶ ἧττον ἐν ὑγρότητι καὶ ξηρότητι. *Loc. Aff. 3.6. K.VIII:* 163, 6–10.

137

Sleep in Galen

Just like sleep and insomnia are produced by a mixture exceeded in the amount of humidity in the former, and dryness in the latter; in the same way, on these particular qualities [depend] the seriousness or mildness of insomnia and [the depth or lightness of] sleep, for they correspond to the increased or reduced amount of humidity and dryness.

Clearly, Galen's system contemplates this perfect continuum between antithetical symptoms, which are correlated with opposed qualities. The same rationale underpins the polarity that contrasts *lethargy* with *phrenitis*. Consistently throughout his works, the former is hypoactive and caused by the coldest and wettest mixtures, whereas the latter is hyperactive and the result of the hottest and driest *kraseis:*

... φρενῖτις μὲν ξηρὸν καὶ θερμόν ἐστι νόσημα, καὶ διὰ τοῦτο ταῖς πρακτικαῖς ἐνεργείαις εὐρωστότατον· ὁ δὲ λήθαργος ἄρρωστον, ὑγρότητι δαψιλεῖ τε καὶ ψυχρᾷ... *Caus. Symp. III.10. K.VII:* 259, 18; 260, 1–3.

... *phrenitis* is a dry and hot disease and this is why it is particularly strong in active functions [hyperactive]. *Lethargy* is weak [in active functions, that is, hypoactive] due to abundance of humidity and coldness. ...

Although Galen does not explicitly link these phenomena to the quantitative aspect of his humoural theory, he does illustrate his explanations with the same examples as those he had used to explore the gradability of the theory. Therefore, it is not unreasonable to think that – also in this regard – he did consider the levels of consciousness to be parallel to the degrees of the qualities: *somnolenta igitur, quantum ad praesens, ipsis litargicis insidet, insomnem vero, que freneticis supervenit, temptandum distinguere.* ('Therefore, somnolent [*kataphora*] – which determines the degree of *lethargy* itself – should be distinguished from sleepless [*kataphora*], which can befall *phrenitic* patients').[5] In other words, impaired consciousness (*kataphora*) can manifest with symptoms that extend from sleep – at the hypoactive end of the spectrum – all the way through to wakefulness, with a whole range of intermediate states. In such states, presumably, the degrees of heat, coldness, moistness and dryness determine the severity of the delirium or the depth of the sleep, which are ultimately two sides of the same coin.

[5] *Hipp. Com. CMG V.9.2; 3.1:* 188, 34–6. *K.VII:* 656.

138

From a less pathophysiological point of view, it is interesting to place this concept of correlations between depths of sleep and seriousness of ailments within a broader context and amid the non-medical discourses. There is an explicit philosophical formulation in Aristotle's *Generation of animals*:

ὕπνος εἶναι δοκεῖ τὴν φύσιν τῶν τοιούτων, οἷον τοῦ ζῆν καὶ τοῦ μὴ ζῆν μεθόριον, καὶ οὔτε μὴ εἶναι παντελῶς ὁ καθεύδων οὔτ᾽ εἶναι. *GA. LCL V*: 778b.

Sleep seems to have this very nature: it is like a boundary between not living and living; for somebody asleep is neither being nor completely not-being.

If we consider that death is often the end stage of serious illnesses, and that according to these doctors becoming progressively sick manifests by becoming progressively drowsy, one can see how these closely connected ideas have possibly interacted and interfered with each other. Indeed, the liminality of sleep between life and death seems to have been deeply ingrained in ancient discourses (well beyond archaic epic poetry). It penetrated medicine to such an extent that even Celsus, who did not conceive a progression in the levels of consciousness, still regarded sleep as a sign of imminent death: *eadem mors denuntiatur ... ubi adsidue dormit* ('Death itself is announced ... when one sleeps uninterruptedly').[6]

To sum up, the way in which these authors tackled sleep illustrates how strict definitions and clear boundaries sometimes obscure phenomena, rather than help to explain them. Celsus' strict separation between wakefulness and sleep prevented him from considering intermediate conditions and stages that were present in other contemporary treatises. Furthermore, although he was interested – as most other post-Hellenistic sources – in the relationship between perceptions and reality, he only discussed the topic in connection with delirium but not with sleep (as Aretaeus and Galen did), thereby leaving out questions about the reality of dreams. In a similar manner, Galen's clear distinction between health and disease did not allow

---

[6] *Med. II: 6, 5.* In the Latin tradition, Pliny the Elder went a step even further by equating normal healthy sleep with death: *quid quod aestimatione nocturnae quietis dimidio quisque spatio vitae suae vivit, pars aequa morti similis exigitur?* ('What about the fact that by considering our nightly rest, everybody lives half of the time of his life, whereas an equal part is taken away by a state resembling death?' *Nat. Hist. VII.50, 167*: 618, 1–3).

him to see the gradual transition between both stages. He seems to have clearly understood the progression in the seriousness of illnesses, the related nature of wakefulness and sleep, and even the subtle transition between delirium and drowsiness, but not the link between healthy and disturbed sleep. Paradoxically, both authors took such boundaries for granted and made no effort to define where exactly they set them. Celsus did not explain how to distinguish wakefulness from sleep, nor did Galen clarify where healthy sleep ended and disturbed sleep began. On the contrary, those limits remain as purely theoretical constructions in the texts, which are only self-evident when considering the prototypical extreme situations, but are much less obvious in the intermediate stages.

This lack of explanation is perhaps due to the fact that the exact location of such limits was not established by medicine but by the culture of that time. If – as Williams states – every society organises and schedules the sleep of its members, we can suggest that the medical discourse is only providing explanatory models and solutions (in the form of treatments) for situations where the transgression of social rules is construed as disease.[7] Ultimately, the amount of sleep regarded as normal, the pattern of sleep during night or day and the level of sleepiness acceptable in an interaction are socially regulated conventions.[8] Taking this idea a step further, the whole concept of consciousness that emerges from this analysis of sleep could be regarded as the way in which these medical writers accommodated some medical theoretical frameworks to the various non-medical discourses on sleep available in their time and place.

Galen's approach to HOFs, the mind and their terminology

Unlike the previous authors, where the idea of mind and the organisation of HOFs had to be deduced from hints in the descriptions, Galen was very explicit about it and delimited a systematic, coherent and consistent division of the different domains involved in the workings of the mind:

---

[7] Williams (2008: 637).   [8] Worthman and Melby (2002: 90).

... τὰς ψυχικὰς [ἐνεργείας] ... τέμνοντες εἴς τε τὰς αἰσθητικὰς καὶ τὰς κινητικὰς καὶ τρίτας τὰς ἡγεμονικὰς ... πάλιν ἑκάστην τῶν εἰρημένων διαιροῦμεν εἰς τὰς ἐν αὐτῇ διαφοράς. ἡ μὲν οὖν αἰσθητικὴ τῆς ψυχῆς ἐνέργεια πέντε τὰς πάσας ἔχει διαφοράς: ὁρατ<ικ>ήν, καὶ ὀσφρητ<ικ>ήν, καὶ γευστ<ικ>ήν, καὶ ἀκουστ<ικ>ήν, καὶ ἁπτ<ικ>ήν. ἡ δὲ κινητικὴ τὸ μὲν προσεχὲς ὄργανον ἓν ἔχει καὶ τὸν τρόπον αὐτοῦ τῆς κινήσεως ἕνα ... ἡ λοιπὴ δὲ ἐνέργεια τῆς ψυχῆς ἡ κατ' αὐτὸ τὸ ἡγεμονικὸν εἴς τε τὸ φανταστικὸν καὶ διανοητικὸν καὶ μνημονευτικὸν διαιρεῖται. *Symp. Diff. CMG (G).3*: 216, 19–20; 218, 1–6, 7–9. *K.VII*: 55–6.

... Having separated the psychic [activities] into perception, movement and thirdly, authoritative (*hêgemonikas*) [activities] ... we will divide them, again, into classificatory categories within each. The perceptual activity of the *psuchê* has five sub-categories: sight, smell, taste, hearing and touch. The motor [activity] has a single organ attached, and the form of its movement is also one ... The remaining activities of the *psuchê* – which are controlled by the *hêgemonikon* (authoritative part) – [can be classified] into imagination (*phantastikon*), intellect (*dianoêtikon*) and memory (*mnêmoneutikon*).[9]

In this passage, Galen is establishing clear boundaries of what constitutes 'the psychic', what its sub-divisions are and what are their corresponding activities or functions. It is within these theoretical limits that he will later discuss all the conditions that we nowadays consider as wakeful and drowsy impaired consciousness. We could be tempted to regard the activities of the *hêgemonikon* as similar to our current medical idea of consciousness.[10] However, other texts present minor variations in terminology and some nuances in the concepts, which prevent such a correspondence. In a more philosophical work, for instance, Galen states that ἡ λογιστικὴ ψυχὴ δυνάμεις ἔχει πλείους, αἴσθησιν καὶ μνήμην καὶ σύνεσιν ἑκάστην τε τῶν ἄλλων ('the rational (*logistikê*) *psuchê* has several capacities: perception, memory and understanding (*sunesin*) of each of the others').[11] When comparing the two extracts there appears to be some overlap and

---

9 For the translation of *hêgemonikon* as authoritative part, I have followed Johnston (2006: 188 n. 20).
10 Particularly when Galen offers alternative designations to it: καὶ τὸ ἡγεμονικὸν, καὶ τὸ ἡγεμονοῦν, καὶ τὸ ἡγούμενον καὶ τὸ δεσπόζον καὶ τὸ ἄρχον καὶ τὸ λογιζόμενον καὶ τὸ νοοῦν καὶ τὸ φρονοῦν ('the governing part, as well as the part with authority, the part that guides, rules, leads, calculates, thinks, and the part that has understanding', *PHP. CMG II.5*: 144, 5–6. *K.V*: 258).
11 *QAM Teubner 2*: 34, 23–5. *K.IV*: 771. Because this passage summarises what Galen had said previously about the capacities, I interpret that ἑκάστην τε τῶν ἄλλων refers to perceptions and memory, thereby implying that the rational soul has an understanding of what has been perceived and what can be recalled.

simplification between what he had defined as 'psychic activities' and what he is designating as 'the capacities of the rational *psuchê*'. In yet another treatise the *hêgemonikon* is the site where ἐπιστήμης τε καὶ δόξης ἁπάσης τε διανοήσεως ('knowledge (*epistêmê*), all the judgement (*doxa*) and intellect (*dianoêsis*) are to be found'),[12] and later on he states that αἱ μὲν τοῦ λογιστικοῦ τῆς ψυχῆς ἐνέργειαι καλείσθωσαν ἡγεμονικαὶ ('the activities of the rational (*logistikou*) part of the *psuchê* should be called *hêgemonikai* [that is, belonging to the authoritative part]').[13] Ultimately, although there are some discrepancies concerning what belongs to the rational *psuchê* in general and to the *hêgemonikon* in particular,[14] it seems that Galen is grouping together some HOFs, most of which are nowadays considered to belong in the sphere of consciousness.[15] Moreover, it could be argued that in this sense he remained remarkably consistent throughout his work. He considered all the diseases that affect these *psychikai/ hêgemonikai energeiai*, or the *logistikon tês psuchês* to be related,[16] and he offered a comprehensive catalogue of them in his treatise *On the distinction of symptoms*:

καὶ τοίνυν αἱ βλάβαι τῶν αἰσθητικῶν ἐνεργειῶν κοιναὶ μὲν ἁπασῶν ἀναισθησίαι τινές εἰσιν, ἢ δυσαισθησίαι ... καὶ πρὸς τούτοις ἔτι δύο ἐξαίρετα, τὸ μὲν ἀγρυπνία, τὸ δὲ κῶμα ... τῶν δ᾽ αὖ κινητικῶν ἐνεργειῶν ἀκινησία μὲν καὶ δυσκινησία τὰ πρῶτα συμπτώματα ... ἐπειδὰν ... ἐμπροσθότονός τε καὶ ὀπισθότονος καὶ τέτανος ... ἐπιληψία ... καὶ ἀποπληξία ἢ παντὸς τοῦ σώματος παράλυσις ἅμα ταῖς ἡγεμονικαῖς ἐνεργείαις ... ἐφεξῆς δ᾽ ἂν εἴη τὰς τῶν ἡγεμονικῶν ἐνεργειῶν βλάβας διελθεῖν, καὶ πρώτης γε τῆς φανταστικῆς. ἔστι δὲ καὶ ταύτης ... ὃ δὲ κάρος καὶ κατάληψις ... παραφροσύνη ... τὸ δὲ οἷον ἐλλιπὴς καὶ ἄτονος [κίνησις], ὡς ἐν κώμασί τε καὶ ληθάργοις ... καὶ μέν γε καὶ αὐτῆς τῆς διανοητικῆς ἐνεργείας ... ἄνοια ... μωρία τε καὶ μώρωσις ... παραφροσύνη. *Symp. Diff. 3 K.VII*: 56, 58–60.

The damages common to all the perceptual activities are certain *anaesthesiai* or *dusaesthesiai* ... apart from these, there are also two special ones: sleeplessness and *kôma* ... Again, the main symptoms of the motor activities are immobility (*akinesia*) and *duskinesia* ... then, *emprosthotonos*, *opisthotonos* and tetanus, ...

---

[12] *Loc. Aff. CAM II.10*: 372, 22. *K.VIII*: 126.   [13] *Loc. Aff. 3.6. K.VIII*: 163, 2–3.

[14] We have seen yet another similar though not identical division of activities in *The art of medicine* (*Ars. Med. CUF 6.9*: 290, 11–14. *K.I*: 322).

[15] McDonald (2014: 139–40) has also noted some divergence and some coincidence in the verbs that Galen chose to describe the specific activities of the *hêgemonikon* in *On the affected parts* as compared to *On the doctrines of Hippocrates and Plato*.

[16] Galen sometimes uses these terms interchangeably, although according to the previous explanation one is subordinated to the other.

epilepsy . . . and *apoplexy* or simultaneous paralysis of the whole body and the activities of the *hêgemonikon* [authoritative part] . . . Subsequently, the damages to the *hêgemonikon* [itself] should be discussed, and firstly those that affect the imagination (*phantastikon*). Amongst them are . . . torpor (*karos*) and *catalepsy* . . . delirium (*paraphrosunê*) . . . [and] something akin to a defective [movement] lacking tone, as in *kômas* and *lethargies* . . . And among those [damages] that affect the intellectual activities (*dianoêtikon*), there are . . . mindlessness (*anoia*) . . . folly (*môria*) and foolishness (*môrôsis*) . . . [and] delirium (*paraphrosunê*).

Although there are other classifications throughout the corpus with minor variations, as well as certain conditions that are not mentioned here (which Galen nonetheless considered to belong in this group),[17] there is consistency in terms of the anatomical and physio-pathological understanding. All these conditions affect the brain (because it is the seat of the rational soul), and they all occur as a consequence of an imbalance in the *krasis*,[18] namely, an approach with evident advantages in terms of therapeutic conduct, for it explained diseases in a way that enabled Galenic medicine to successfully treat them.

Regarding the organisation of the mind, Galen's fragmentation of the HOFs blurred several distinctions that we now make (because they were irrelevant to his therapeutic approach). Thus, by describing all these conditions as affections of the *psuchê*,[19] and classifying them according to the type of psychic activity disturbed (perception, motion or ruling part) and the kind of compromise (complete, partial or deviant), the edges between impaired consciousness (wakeful or drowsy) and mental illnesses become fuzzy, for they are both diseases where the intellectual

---

[17] τὰ μὲν οὖν πάθη τὰ ψυχικὰ φόβοι τέ εἰσιν ἐξαιφνίδιοι καὶ σφοδροί . . . αἵ τ᾽ ἐναντίαι τοῖς φόβοις ἡδοναὶ μέγισται ('The psychic affections are sudden and excessive fears, as well as their opposite, namely, great pleasures', *MM.* XII.5: 370, 3–5. *K.X*: 841).

[18] In this respect, Devinant (2020) offers a similar idea from a different perspective. In his search for a delimitation of Galenic psychic disturbances, he also highlights the anatomical and qualitative dimensions of Galen's analysis (127–8), and the focus on the brain as the seat of these conditions (137–42). The problem with framing them as 'psychic disturbances' and not impaired consciousness is that Devinant's approach leaves out sleep and fainting, which also seemed to be connected to these conditions in the Galenic conceptions.

[19] Not surprisingly, several scholars have addressed Galen's understanding of madness while discussing his ideas on the soul: Pigeaud (2008: 562–83), Jouanna (2013: 97–118), Nutton (2013b: 119–28) and Boudon-Millet (2013: 129–46).

(*dianoêtikon*) activities of the ruling part of the rational *psuchê* – the *hêgemonikon*[20] – are damaged. Similarly, because the *psuchikai energeiai* are affected in delirium and mental illness, as well as in tetanus, epilepsy and the case of the youth with speechlessness and traumatic paralysis (already mentioned, *Loc. Aff. CMG I.6*: 284, 12–17. *K.VIII*: 50–1), the boundaries between what we now consider as neurological conditions, impaired consciousness and mental illness also become faint. In other words, although Galen subsumed the mental capacities within constructs that are broader than our idea of consciousness, he was able to clinically distinguish cases with impaired consciousness, and he did perceive an abstract notion to be compromised in such situations (albeit a notion comprised of more HOFs than we nowadays consider).

Concerning terminology, as Jouanna has remarked,[21] a parallel passage from *On the causes of symptoms* (*II. 7. K.VII*: 200–4) complements and introduces slight lexical nuances to this list. In this other version Galen calls *môrôsis* what he had previously designated as *anoia*, and defines it as a complete paralysis of the activities of the *dianoêtikon*. The partial impairment of such activities, which he had previously defined as *môria* and *môrôsis*, are now referred to as νάρκαι τοῦ λογισμοῦ τε καὶ τῆς μνήμης ('reason and memory numbness').[22] Interestingly, in this rendering he expands the notion of deliria (*paraphrosunai*) and includes some specific diseases such as *phrenitis*, *mania* and *melancholikai paranoiai*.

Undoubtedly, these passages reveal a fairly standardised and rather concise vocabulary. Galen's use of terminology, therefore, is more in line with the post-Hellenistic authors than with the Hippocratic doctors, where we found an extensive use of partial synonymy. Although there was a certain instability (for example, between *anoia/môrôsis* when tackling the diseases of the *dianoêtikon*), in the last passages,

---

[20] These diseases affect the rational soul but do not alter its leading role within the human being. A whole other group of conditions, where the spirited and the desiderative soul prevail over the rational one are discussed in *On the doctrines of Hippocrates and Plato* (*PHP IV.6. CMG*: 278, 5–9. *K.V*: 412–13). Unlike the descriptions that we nowadays frame as character traits or ethical behaviours, in conditions that can be equated with impaired consciousness the rational soul tends to be compromised, but still in control over the others.

[21] Jouanna (2013: 109).   [22] *Caus. Symp. II, 7. K.VII*: 201, 16.

his vocabulary reminds us of Aretaeus': *paraphrosunê* seems to be the most common word for delirium (even if *parakoptô* is exceptionally used to describe similar phenomena).[23] *Paranoia* in the comment on *melancholia* was used to designate the specific kind of delusion that characterised that condition. Finally, *paralêrêsis* – as in Aretaeus – is the word chosen to talk about the mental disturbance of old age (what we would nowadays call dementia): διὰ τί τοίνυν εἰς ἔσχατον γῆρας ἀφικνούμενοι παρελήρησαν οὐκ ὀλίγοι τῆς τοῦ γέρως ἡλικίας ἀποδεδειγμένης εἶναι ξηρᾶς; οὐ διὰ τὴν ξηρότητα φήσομεν ἀλλὰ διὰ τὴν ψυχρότητα ('Why do most of those who reach extreme old age act foolishly (*parelêrêsan*), if old age has been demonstrated to be dry? We shall reply, not due to the dryness but to the coldness').[24] Once again, there is a humoural correlate that will guide the specific treatment of this clinical condition.

---

[23] Devinant (2020, 112–14) offers a thorough analysis of Galen's use of this term.
[24] *QAM Teubner* 5: 47, 18–21. *K.IV*: 786.

CHAPTER 11

SLEEP AND THE MIND: AN OVERVIEW OF IDEAS THAT DID NOT CHANGE

By framing sleep as a form of impaired consciousness, a common feature emerged in all the sources, namely, its ambiguous status in relation to various dichotomous oppositions. Indeed, when talking about dormancy, authors seem to be constantly navigating the tensions between health and disease,[1] wakefulness and unconsciousness, and in certain cases, even between life and death. Medical writers tended to be torn – to a greater or lesser extent – by some of these oppositions, and they struggled to locate sleep at a determined point between the polar extremes of one or several of these antithetical pairs.

Closely related to the previous finding is another feature that pervades the different periods: the perceived sense of gradual transition between the antithetic extremes, which brings us back to the questions about limits. Whether such extremes are envisaged as a continuous spectrum or as a sequence of discrete stages, the manner in which most of the authors (except for Celsus) discussed sleep points towards ideas of progression, rather than abrupt changes from one state to its opposite. Understandably, if biological processes are gradual, establishing boundaries between intermediate categories is not straightforward, for they have fuzzy edges. When juxtaposing these ancient medical ideas with our existing sociological understandings about sleep,[2] one can see that it is often the social conventions – such as what is acceptable and what is not – that establish clearer boundaries, thereby exemplifying a situation where sociological discourse has an influence over science.

---

[1] Given the great popularity of the cult of Asklepios and the ritual of incubation in his temples throughout all antiquity, another surprising coincidence in all these texts is the complete lack of reference to sleep and dreams as healing processes in this context. Because there are no allusions to the practices at the *Asklepieia* among the medical writers that I am analysing, and due to the scope of the topic, I have chosen not to include it in my discussion. (A comprehensive study of this topic can be found in Renberg, 2017.)

[2] Taylor (1993), Williams (2008) and Asmis (2016).

Concerning the terminology, from a historical perspective, there is an evident quantitative shrinkage in the vocabulary of delirium from the Hippocratic authors onwards. The abundant glossaries and attempts at shedding light on the meaning of each term[3] suggest that those authors had used a larger terminology than their successors to talk about delirium. This reduction might further support the idea of partial synonymy. Ultimately, the Hippocratic corpus was written by many authors from different parts of the Greek world, and it is understandable that they utilised varied terms to talk about similar realities. On the other hand, the fact that the later authors that we looked at required (to describe similar cases) only a few of those terms might indicate that a more limited number of words was sufficient because many of them expressed similar symptoms.

In terms of the organisation and workings of the mind, the previous analysis has yielded other elements that remained constant throughout the different periods and authors, which points towards a general common understanding of impaired consciousness. To be sure, medical writers related the condition to certain abstract notions that they deemed to be compromised (whether we call them the mind, HOFs or a rudimentary idea of consciousness) and struggled to link – in a clear example of tension between theory and clinic – such concepts to the symptoms found in their patients. This becomes particularly evident when considering the extensive use of phrasal terms and their similar structure (a noun head with an HOF and a determiner in the semantic field of 'damage' or 'compromise'). These lexicalisations, therefore, support the hypothesis that an underlying intellectual construct was shared, regardless of the specific nuances that each author gave it (in the case of Galen I have not mentioned any phrasal term, but the underlying constructs are explicitly described).

The tension that emerges from the interaction between these theoretical concepts and the actual clinical findings reflects how these authors – implicitly or explicitly – conceived the relationship between mind and body, cognition and behaviour, thereby characterising the singularity of each medical writer's understanding. It is, certainly, this tension – which each author resolved in a different

---

[3] di Benedetto's (1986: 43–7), Pigeaud's (1987: 15–19) and Thumiger's (2013: 63–81).

manner – that conditioned the changes or evolution in the idea of consciousness discussed throughout the analysis.

Finally, these theoretical constructs also illustrate the important degree of abstract reflection that all these authors reached, which they defended even to the detriment of some observational evidence. Indeed, these rudimentary notions of consciousness – first described with various terms by the Hippocratic texts – were powerful enough to organise most of the later theorisations of delirium, sleep and intermediate states that we have been discussing. Accordingly, the post-Hellenistic authors were happy to sacrifice coherence and consistency in their pathophysiological explanations but preserved these embryonic ideas of consciousness, whereas Galen devised a coherent anatomical and pathophysiological system, but could easily overlook some contemporary nosological classifications in order to preserve these constructs. In other words, the specificities about the way in which each of the authors fragmented or grouped the HOFs – that is, the particularities of each one's rudimentary notion of consciousness – determined the clinical differences that they were able to see, as well as those that remained obscure.

PART III

FAINTING

CHAPTER 12

GENERAL OVERVIEW OF TOTAL LOSS OF CONSCIOUSNESS

Contemporary medicine conceives total loss of consciousness as a global alteration of brain activity. It can have a neurological origin such as in seizures, strokes, head trauma or other aetiologies that ultimately affect the central nervous system (intoxications, infections, liver conditions, etc., where the damage is mediated by substances that compromise neurons). Alternatively, total loss of consciousness can be caused by impaired cerebral blood flow. Such cases can be the result of significant haemorrhages; but they can also be transient and self-limited episodes, which we define as 'syncope'[1] or, less technically, swoons and fainting. The latter are usually preceded by dizziness, light-headedness and sometimes visual and auditory disturbances (pre-syncope). Three main varieties of syncopes are usually recognised: those that are neurally mediated (or vasovagal), which are due to a transient impairment of the autonomic nervous system; postural (or orthostatic) hypotension, in which the blood pressure drops when individuals stand up (and hence they faint), owing to a permanent disorder in the autonomic nervous system; and finally, cardiac syncope, secondary to arrhythmia or a structural heart disease (mainly valvulopathy or ischaemia). In contemporary times vasovagal syncopes are epidemiologically the most frequent and are typically triggered by strong emotions, pain and – often – the sight of blood. Accompanying signs can include pallor, sweating (*diaphoresis*), cardiac symptoms (especially palpitations), gastric symptoms (such as nausea and vomiting), hypoventilation and sudden muscle contractions (*myoclonus*). These episodes are sometimes described as near-death experiences.[2] This chapter

---

[1] I will use 'syncope' to refer to our current medical understanding of the phenomenon, and the Greek transliteration, *sunkopê*, to refer to an ancient nosological entity that probably emerged in the Hellenistic period.

[2] Freeman (2011: chapter 20) offers a detailed and in-depth description of current medical ideas on syncope.

analyses the way in which ancient doctors explained and treated these kinds of conditions.

In order to talk about total loss of consciousness, compounds of *psuchê* have often been used in the ancient Greek medical tradition, and compounds of *anima* in Latin. As we shall see, there is a distinction among most ancient medical writers (in some it is more subtle than in others) between two forms of this prototypical presentation: firstly, one that authors perceived to be related to the soul; and secondly, one framed as an eminently physical condition, where bodily symptoms predominated.

The discussion, therefore, will address what Helen King has denominated as 'common to body and soul'. The tension between these two elements constituted a central topic of debate among philosophers in antiquity in terms of what pertained to the body, what to the soul and what was shared by both.[3] Closely related to this discussion is the debate concerning the authors' support for either instrumentalism or materialism (the former being the idea of the body as simply an instrument of the soul, and the latter as the soul depending completely on the effect of bodily substances).[4] The above-mentioned two forms of understanding of total loss of consciousness will allow us to explore the extent to which medical writers engaged in these controversies, and how they negotiated between these opposite extremes.

In other words, the complete disruption of HOFs that occurred when a patient fainted – where wakefulness, cognition, perception and movement (that is, alertness, connectedness, responsiveness) were temporarily suppressed – can provide some clues about notions held by these medical writers, which went well beyond their ideas around consciousness. Indeed, implicit in those explanations are their perceptions concerning the soul, its relation to the body and occasionally, even their views on the boundaries between life and death.

---

[3] King (2006: 3).

[4] There are two particularly interesting recent analyses about this debate in antiquity. Bartos (2015: 184–6) proposes an instrumental relation between body and soul in the Hippocratic *On regimen* (while rejecting dualistic interpretations of the treatise), and Devinant's (2020: 35–9) starting point for his inquiry about Galen is the apparent contradiction between *The capacities of the soul follow the mixtures of the body* and *On the use of parts* regarding the debate between instrumentalism and materialism.

It should be emphasised, however, that in no way does the following analysis pretend to be an exhaustive philosophical study on ancient psychology. As stated in the Preface, it will only address the notion of the soul as far as it is relevant to understanding these medical writers' stances on impaired consciousness and it will only touch upon extra-medical sources (mainly philosophical) whenever they are key to illuminating some of these authors' claims.

CHAPTER 13

THE HIPPOCRATIC CORPUS AND TOTAL LOSS OF CONSCIOUSNESS

Two forms of losing consciousness among the Hippocratic doctors

Throughout several Hippocratic treatises, fainting is often construed using terms that etymologically suggest separation of, lack of or a diminished *psuchê* (*leipopsuchiê, apsuchiê, oligopsuchiê*, etc.).[1] Such are the cases of bilious women who faint (*oligopsuchiê empiptei*)[2] because their *menses* are retained; or cases of swoons when lifting from the seat; namely, examples of what we would nowadays frame as an orthostatic syncope. In *Epidemics VII*, a patient fainted (*eleipopsuxei*) on the ninth day of his disease ἐπὶ θῶκον ἀναστὰς ('when standing up from the chair').[3]

Unlike descriptions of delirium where etymology was completely estranged from the meaning of the terms, these writers do seem to have been aware of the lexical components involved in the words they used, because in their view the soul was a key factor in this syndrome. Accordingly, the author of *On diseases I* seems to conceive fainting as a separation of the *psuchê*:

ὅσοισιν ἢ ἐκψύχουσιν δεῖ τι ὠφελῆσαι . . . οὗτοι μὲν οἱ καιροὶ ὀξέες, καὶ οὐκ ἀρκέει ὀλίγῳ ὕστερον· ἀπόλλυνται γὰρ οἱ πολλοὶ ὀλίγῳ ὕστερον . . . ὅ τι ἄν τις πρὸ τοῦ τὴν ψυχὴν μεθεῖναι ὠφελήσῃ, τοῦθ' ἅπαν ἐν καιρῷ ὠφέλησεν. *Morb. I. LCL 5*: 96, 4; 7–12.

One needs to help those who faint (*ekpsuchousin*) ... These opportunities are urgent, and a little later is not good enough, for most patients die a little later ... whatever help one can offer before the *psuchê* breaks free is offered at the exactly right opportunity.

---

[1] *Leipothumiê* is also used interchangeably with these terms. However, unlike the compounds of *psuchê* – all of which imply loss of consciousness – only this compound of *thumos* is associated with swoons. The others have different connotations: the author of *On ancient medicine* uses *apsuchiê* to talk about fainting but *dusthumiê* to convey the idea of mood alterations (*VM 10.4*: 86). Thumiger (2017: 349–50) presents other examples – *oxuthumiê, euthumiê* – where these compounds are used to describe emotional states.
[2] *Mul. I. LCL 8*: 36, 13.   [3] *Epid. VII. CUF 84.5*: 99, 25–6.

The previous example implies that for this author *ekpsuchô* evoked the idea of a release of the *psuchê*. Because the separation could become irreversible, thereby leading to death, his idea of soul suggests some kind of life force and warrants immediate help before the soul breaks free for good.[4] My interpretation questions Thumiger's point of view that the idea of the *psuchê* was only relevant in very few texts.[5] On the contrary, it implies that it was present in several of these authors' idea of swoons. In the previous example, it seems that the medical writer regarded fainting as a partial, temporary and reversible separation of the *psuchê*, compatible with a near-death experience.[6]

Not surprisingly, in these near-death experiences the Hippocratic doctors paid particular attention to respiration: in a patient who had fainted (that is, someone non-alert, disconnected, unresponsive), breathing provided some evidence that could give the observer a valuable clue as to whether the patient was dead or had only momentarily lost consciousness. This is advised by the author of *On regimen in acute diseases B*: καταμανθάνειν δὲ καὶ ἐν τῆσιν ἐξαναστάσεσιν, εἰ λειποθυμέει ἢ εἰ τοῦ πνεύματος εὐφορίη αὐτὸν ἔχει ('one should observe carefully whether the patient faints or breathes easily as he stands up').[7] Similar examples can be found elsewhere (*Acut. Sp. 23. LCL*: 248, 16–17 and *Epid. V. CUF 2, 2–3*: 3, 1–5).[8] Polycrates' physician is even more explicit when describing a specific type of breathing characteristic of fainting (we would nowadays define it as 'agonal' or 'gasping' respiration):

... πνεῦμα μέτριον, ἔστι δ᾽ ὅτε καὶ ἅλες ἑλκύσας πάλιν ἀθρόον ἐξέπνει, ὥσπερ ὑπ᾽ ἀψυχίης, ἢ ὡς ἂν διὰ πνίγους πορευθεὶς ἐν σκιῇ καθεζόμενος ὥς τις ἀναπνεύσειε. *Epid. VII. CUF 1, 6*: 48, 12–15.

---

4 Note the difference with the role of the soul during sleep. As Bartos (2015: 203–4) has remarked, in *On regimen* the soul becomes more independent from the body during sleep but it still cooperates with it and always moves within its limits; it does not separate from it.

5 Thumiger (2017: 405).

6 From a rhetorical point of view, this nosological treatise is exemplifying, in a practical context, an idea that *On the art* and *On breaths* had postulated about medicine (which was shared by different authors of the corpus); namely, that the mission of this group of practitioners was to oppose disease and death: ... νούσων ... θανάτου· πᾶσι γὰρ τούτοισιν ἄντικρυς ἡ ἰητρική ('... diseases ... death. To all this things medicine is opposed', *Flat. CUF I.2*: 103, 3–4).

7 *Acut. Sp. LCL 22*: 248, 5–6.

8 The second author explains that because the patient was not breathing, he seemed (*edokei*) to be dead.

... moderate breathing: after drawing in a big gasp [of air], he would exhale it again suddenly, like somebody [who had] fainted, or like one who sits in the shade to recover his breath after walking in the heat.

Apparently, in this transient separation of the *psuchê*, breathing continues throughout the whole swoon, and it is this very condition that reveals to the doctor whether the fainting patient still lived or if he had passed away.

A final remark with regards to this form of describing total loss of consciousness concerns its fuzzy edges with wakeful impaired consciousness. It is suggested in a case where orthostatic syncope is considered as an early sign of delirium (*paraphrosunê*): τοῦ πνεύματος ἀπορίη, ἢ διαναστὰς ἐπὶ θρόνον ἢ αὐτοῦ ἐν τῇ κλίνῃ ἦν ἀψυχίη ἐγγένηται ('difficulty in breathing or if the patient faints while he is standing up from a seat or from his bed').[9] In other words the momentary departure of the soul can presage conditions where the mind is unsound.

On the other hand, the Hippocratic doctors also found another way of describing total loss of consciousness, in which the soul does not seem to be involved. Head trauma, which we could even nowadays easily relate to suddenly becoming unconscious, is described in the following way: δῖνός τε ἔλαβε καὶ σκότος, καὶ ἐκαρώθη καὶ κατέπεσεν ('he suffered vertigo, blacked out (*elabe skotos*), became drowsy (*ekarôthê*) and fell down').[10] Note the assimilation of total loss of consciousness with drowsiness for this author through the verb *karoô*. As a matter of fact, instead of conceiving this sudden episode as a single concept, the writer seems to be describing concurrent, yet separate clinical symptoms.

The author of *Diseases of women II* offers a similar enumeration when describing what appears to be a swoon:

ὅταν ὑστέρη πνίγῃ, πνεῦμα δὲ σεύηται ἅλες ἄνω, καὶ βάρος ἔχῃ, καὶ γνώμη καταπλὴξ, ἀναυδίη, περίψυξις, πνεῦμα προσπταῖον, ὄμματα ἀμαλδύνηται. *Mul. II. LCL.92*: 424, 14–17.

When the womb suffocates, the air is driven upwards in gasps, torpor is experienced and the *gnômê* is struck. Speechlessness, shivering, laboured breathing and weakened eyes.

---

[9] *Acut. Sp. LCL 23*: 248, 16–17.   [10] *VC. CMG 14.5*: 82, 12–13.

Again, the excerpt presents a periphrastic list of symptoms that resemble a swoon. There is a cognitive compromise, which is referred to through the phrasal term 'struck *gnômê*', and a strong emphasis on the bodily symptoms, particularly the attention to breathing (which was also present in the cases of *leipothumiê* and *apsuchiê* mentioned above) and the insistence in both excerpts on the blurring of vision (ὄμματα ἀμαλδύνηται and ἔλαβε καὶ σκότος).[11] The cases of *apoplexy* – as Walshe has accurately remarked – are also conditions with 'sudden loss of consciousness, paralysis, and collapse'.[12] We have already seen an example when discussing HOFs, where the description of the author of *On glands* follows the same pattern of concurrent and simultaneous separate symptoms: movement disturbances, speechlessness, suffocation and a bewildered *nous*.[13]

It seems as though where we nowadays simply perceive total loss of consciousness, the Hippocratic authors could perceive two subtly different realities. One was described using compounds of *psuchê* or *thumos*, which was conceived as a near-death experience; the second was a concurrent accumulation of physical losses that eventually led to passing out. This very nuance might be at the origin of the notion of *sunkopê*, a condition (also designated as *cardiacum*) probably described as a disease in its own right at some point during the Hellenistic period (it appears in most post-Hellenistic treatises, but is never mentioned as such in the Hippocratic corpus).

An all-encompasing Hippocratic *psuchê*

Several Hippocratic texts portray the *psuchê* as an all-encompassing concept which subsumed cognitive and bodily functions. We have already seen that the author of *On breaths* considered *hai psuchai* to

---

[11] Perhaps there is a Homeric influence to it. Dying and fainting in the *Iliad* are often expressed as the *psuchê* or the *thumos* abandoning the hero while – at the same time – darkness, mist or the night itself blind him. Some examples are: θυμὸν ἀποπνείων ... τὸν δὲ σκότος ὄσσε κάλυψε (*Il. IV*: 524–6); τὸν δ' ἔλιπε ψυχή, κατὰ δ' ὀφθαλμῶν κέχυτ' ἀχλύς (*Il. V*: 696); τὴν δὲ κατ' ὀφθαλμῶν ἐρεβεννὴ νὺξ ἐκάλυψεν ... ἀπὸ δὲ ψυχὴν ἐκάπυσσε (*Il. XXII*: 366–7).

[12] Walshe (2016: 99).

[13] ὁ νόος ἀφραίνει, καὶ ὁ ἐγκέφαλος σπᾶται καὶ ἕλκει τὸν ὅλον ἄνθρωπον, ἐνίοτε δ' οὐ φωνέει καὶ πνίγεται, ἀποπληξίῃ τῷ πάθει τοὔνομα (the *nous* acts irrationally and the brain suffers spasms which drag along the whole body; sometimes he is speechless and chokes: the name of the affection is *apoplexy*) (*Glan. 12.2. Brill(C).*: 76, 13–15).

contain *phronêmata*,[14] while the author of *On regimen* talked initially about *phronêsis* as a condition of the *psuchê*,[15] whereas later on he expanded the idea. In book 4, the *psuchê* is said to renounce its own *dianoia* during wakefulness in favour of the body – which suggests that it contains a *dianoia* – but once the body falls asleep, it wakes up and γινώσκει πάντα, καὶ ὁρῇ τε τὰ ὁρατὰ καὶ ἀκούει τὰ ἀκουστά, βαδίζει, ψαύει, λυπεῖται, ἐνθυμεῖται ('recognises everything, sees what can be seen, hears what can be heard, walks, touches, suffers, assesses').[16] The relevance of this comprehensiveness of the soul is that it is responsible for cognition, perception, motion, emotion and reason. Because this Hippocratic *psuchê* is active during sleep, present during wakeful life – even if it is τῷ σώματι ὑπηρετέουσα ('subjected to the body')[17] – and its absence means death, I disagree with the idea suggested by some scholars that this model presents strong Homeric echoes.[18]

Beyond the sources commented on above, there is another Hippocratic text, *On humours* (a disjointed miscellany of observations about various medical topics),[19] which offers an even broader catalogue of domains that pertain to the *psuchê*.[20]

ψυχῆς ἀκρασίη ποτῶν καὶ βρωμάτων, ὕπνου, ἐγρηγόρσιος . . . καρτερίη πόνων . . . αἱ μεταβολαὶ ἐξ οἵων ἐς οἷα. ἐκ τῶν ἠθέων, φιλοπονίη ψυχῆς, ἢ ζητῶν, ἢ μελετῶν, ἢ ὁρῶν, ἢ λέγων, ἢ εἴ τι ἄλλο οἷον, λῦπαι, δυσοργησίαι, ἐπιθυμίαι. ἢ τὰ ἀπὸ συγκυρίης λυπήματα γνώμης, ἢ τὰ διὰ τῶν ὀμμάτων, ἢ διὰ τῆς ἀκοῆς καὶ διὰ τῆς γνώμης. οἷα τὰ σώματα, μύλης μὲν τριφθείσης πρὸς ἑωυτήν, ὀδόντες ἡμώδησαν, παρά τε κρημνὸν παριόντι σκέλεα τρέμει, ὅταν τε τῇσι χερσί τις, ὧν μὴ δεῖται, αἴρη αὗται τρέμουσιν. ὄφις ἐξαίφνης ὀφθεὶς χλωρότητα ἐποίησεν. οἱ φόβοι, αἰσχύνη,

[14] *Flat. CUF 14.3*: 122, 8.   [15] *Vict. CMG 1.35.1*: 150, 29.
[16] *Vict. CMG 4.86*, 2: 218, 10–11.   [17] *Vict. CMG 4.86*, 1: 218, 4–5.
[18] Bremmer (1983: 3–66) related this passage to an archaic dual division of the soul into free- and body-souls. However, contrary to his idea of the Homeric 'free-soul' – devoid of psychological attributes and active outside the body during sleep, swoons, trance and death – this *psuchê* has elements of his 'body-soul'. Similarly, the passage is also incompatible with more recent systematisations of archaic Greek thought such as Clarke's (1999: 53–4) tripartite division. In this model, the Homeric *psuchê* is restricted to the domain of death (130), to the imagined life in Hades or to the very moment of dying, when the conscious self departs. Bartos (2015: 165–9), on the contrary, offers a clear description of the way in which the concept changed and progressively acquired the cognitive, intellectual and affective attributes that are apparent in the HC.
[19] Craik (2015: 129–34).
[20] Chapter 9 of this work is extremely obscure, and – as Pigeaud (1981: 42) has suggested – any translation is by necessity an attempt at an interpretation.

ἡδονή, λύπη, ὀργή, τἄλλα τὰ τοιαῦτα. οὕτως ἐνακούει ἑκάστῳ τὸ προσῆκον τοῦ σώματος τῇ πρήξει, ἐν τούτοισιν ἱδρῶτες, καρδίης παλμός, τὰ τοιαῦτα. *Hum. CMG* 9: 168, 3–13.

Belonging to the sphere of the *psuché* are:[21]
  bad balance of drink, nourishment, sleep and wakefulness ... endurance to physical exercise...
  the changes from some conditions to others.
  Among [the changes] in the character: industriousness of the *psuché* when inquiring, exercising, seeing or talking;
    or any other [change] like grief, wrath, desire,
    or the random disturbances of the *gnômê* whether through vision or hearing or through the *gnômê* itself.
  Regarding the bodily [disturbances][22]
      when a mill grinds, the teeth are put on edge;
      when one walks beside a cliff, the legs shake;
      when somebody lifts what he should not with his hands, they tremble;
        the sudden sight of a snake produces pallor;
        fears, shame, grief, pleasure, anger, etc.: the corresponding part of the body reacts to each of them with its own response, which are sweats, heartbeats, etc.

This passage suggests the involvement of the *psuché* in several roles – a few of them already mentioned in *On regimen* (*Vict. CMG 4.86*). Interestingly, after including the *gnômê* within the sphere of the *psuché*,[23] the author focuses on bodily reactions that are beyond rational control, which he also attributes to the *psuché*. This writer seems to be suggesting that the soul governs conscious involuntary reactions, thus further extending the scope of the notion. Perhaps the idea of the *psuché* as 'the most important *life force*', which was common during the fifth century BCE,[24] is associated with this comprehensive collection of functions: it is responsible for the cognitive and perceptual skills, it controls physiological vital capacities (nourishment, sleep, wakefulness),

---

[21] I have arranged the translation as a list, in order to make it easier to visualise my interpretation of the passage and the way in which, I believe, the items are organised.

[22] In my interpretation, unlike Overwien (2014: 212), disturbances are a specific type of change.

[23] Note how *gnômê* – again – seems to convey a notion akin to our idea of cognition, which can be altered by visual and auditory disturbances (hallucinations), as well as by problems within the cognitive capacity itself.

[24] Holmes (2010: 160).

emotions (grief, wrath, desire) and automatic bodily reactions (sweating, breathing, trembling, beating of the heart).

The *psuchê* as the life-giving force

The Hippocratic corpus seems quite consistent regarding the idea of the *psuchê* as a life force, and death is often equated with its definitive separation from the body. We have just discussed a fairly explicit example, where fainting is construed as a temporary separation of the *psuchê* before its final disconnection, when it is too late for treatment.[25] Other Hippocratic texts point in the same direction: in *On internal affections* both descriptions of *typhus* refer to death as ἀφῆκε τὴν ψυχήν ('releasing the *psuchê*').[26] This departure of the *psuchê* or the *thumos* during death does have Homeric echoes;[27] however, these medical writers go a step further. In the *Iliad* it is not implied that the *psuchê* abandons the body during swoons, nor does the departure of the soul during death have a destructive effect in itself on the body.[28] On the contrary, the author of *Epidemics VI* presents a different relationship between body, soul and disease:

ἀνθρώπου ψυχὴ φύεται μέχρι θανάτου· ἢν δὲ ἐκπυρωθῇ ἅμα τῇ νούσῳ καὶ ἡ ψυχή, τὸ σῶμα φέρβεται. (*Epid. VI. LCL 5, 2*: 242, 5–6).

Man's *psuchê* flourishes until death. If it gets consumed by disease, it [the *psuchê*] devours the body.

This diseased *psuchê* seems to have a lethal effect on the body, unlike the Homeric soul that silently moved towards Hades. These cases, therefore, also illustrate a shift in the understanding of the boundaries between life and death, as compared to archaic conceptualisations. In Homer, the *psuchê* left the body through the mouth when wounds were deadly, but it did not harm the body, nor could it come back once it had crossed the fence of teeth. As a matter of fact, the separation of the *psuchê* (and the *thumos*) is almost always synonymous with dying.[29] There are very few exceptions where instead of death, swoons occur, and although the *psuchê* abandons the body, the

---

[25] *Morb. I. LCL 5*: 96, 4; 7–12.   [26] *Int. LCL 39*: 176, 3 and *Int. LCL 40*: 178, 13–14.
[27] According to Clarke (1999: 57), it is the 'dividing line between life and death'.
[28] Clarke (1999: 130).   [29] Barker (2011: 3–11).

character survives because breathing recommences and they come round.[30] As Clarke has remarked, life can be lost through exhalation when the *psuchê* or *thumos* abandon the individual, but it can only be recovered in the form of the *thumos*' vitality being 'sucked into the lungs'.[31] Namely, both concepts are connected with breathing. In the Hippocratic cases of fainting, however, it is probably not so much the 'life soul' represented through the breath that the doctors are carefully observing. Instead, in this medicalised separation of the *psuchê*, breathing is the most obvious clinical sign that distinguishes life from death. Because it is not disrupted during the process, doctors need to notice it in order to know that the individual is alive and further treatment can be used (as also illustrated above, there is a particular kind of breathing characteristic of fainting, which confirms that it is maintained during such episodes).[32]

In summary, considering that delirium (and also sleep) were construed as alterations of the *gnômê*, *sunesis*, *phronêsis* or *nous* (that is, the constructs used by Hippocratic doctors to refer to HOFs) and that such concepts appear to be subsumed within the notion of soul, we could suggest another link between fainting, sleep and delirium. Beyond the shared vocabulary for recovery and the clinical relationship that has already been pointed out, we could also posit a more abstract theoretical connection. It appears that these authors conceived all three presentations as a group of related conditions affecting either the life-giving soul or some capacities subsumed within it. Thus, we could argue that many of these medical writers had a hierarchical understanding of what we nowadays regard as consciousness, in which the cognitive capacities (the mind) were dependent on a more abstract notion, the soul, which in turn enabled life. Following this idea further, impaired consciousness was regarded by them as either a complete or partial affection of the *psuchê*: the soul in its entirety was affected in fainting (sometimes causing near-death experiences), whereas its subordinated cognitive components (*gnômê*, *phronêsis*, *nous*, etc.) were altered or simply changed during delirium and sleep.

---

[30] Such is the case of Sarpedon (τὸν δὲ λίπε ψυχή *Il. V*: 696) and Andromache. The latter faints by gasping out the *psuchê* (ἀπὸ δὲ ψυχὴν ἐκάπυσσε, *Il. XXII*: 467), and comes round when the *thumos* returns to her breast (ἐς φρένα θυμὸς ἀγέρθη, *Il. XXII*: 476).
[31] Clarke (1999: 142).   [32] *Epid. VII. CUF I, 6*: 48, 12–15.

CHAPTER 14

TOTAL LOSS OF CONSCIOUSNESS
IN POST-HELLENISTIC AUTHORS

The post-Hellenistic writers under study responded in various ways to both the Hippocratic and the Hellenistic traditions on total loss of consciousness, and their way of integrating these elements constitutes a clear testimony of their methodology, namely, encyclopaedism in *On medicine*, and lax eclecticism in Aretaeus' work. A common trait that is shared by both authors is the fact that they deepened the Hippocratic dual understanding of this prototypical presentation. For them they were two independent phenomena: either a symptom that appeared in various circumstances – *anima deficit, leipothumiê*, fainting – or an independent disease – *cardiacum, sunkopê*.

Fainting versus *sunkopê*

In Celsus, for example, there seems to be a strong Hippocratic influence in the nomenclature and the presentation of fainting, but a radical difference in the underlying conception of the soul. Similarly, Aretaeus maintained, to a certain extent, the Hippocratic terminology (he used *leipothumiê* and *leipopsuchiê*), but his descriptions were less evidently influenced by the Hippocratic corpus (even if he did not explicitly contradict it). He was particularly concerned with explaining the physiological mechanisms underlying this presentation, in which the soul had limited involvement. The Hellenistic stamp, on the other hand, manifests itself very clearly in the approach to *sunkopê* that both authors express. As we shall see, this affection is regarded as primarily originating in the body, with some kind of alteration in consciousness and descriptions that are suspiciously evocative of our own idea of vasovagal syncope.

Fainting

The terminology that Celsus used to refer to swoons is *anima deficere*. As von Staden has accurately remarked, it is a Latin calque of *leipothumia* and *leipopsuchia*.[1] Also in syntony with the Hippocratic predecessors, fainting was conceived as a separation of the soul. We shall see, however, that Celsus' *anima* is rather different from the Hippocratic *psuchê*.

in capite autem interdum acutus et pestifer morbus est, quem κεφαλαίαν Graeci vocant; cuius notae sunt horror calidus, nervorum resolutio, oculorum caligo, mentis alientatio, vomitus sic ut vox supprimatur, vel sanguinis ex naribus cursus, sic ut corpus frigescat, anima deficiat. *Med. 4.2*: 2.

There is often an acute and destructive disease in the head, which the Greeks call *kephalaia* that presents the following signs: hot shivering; flaccid paralysis; blurred vision; delirium; vomiting, capable of suppressing the voice; or bleeding from the nose, capable of cooling down the body, and of causing fainting.

Suffice here to say that unlike the Hippocratic life force that suddenly and momentarily abandons the body leaving it lifeless, this passage offers a crescendo of symptoms until fainting eventually occurs. In other words, in this disease total loss of consciousness evolves through a progressive loss of capacities – movement, vision, cognition, speech – before the *anima* finally gets to withdraw.

A similar term to designate the same phenomenon is *exanimo*, a calque of the Hippocratic *ekpsuchô*, which also conveys the idea of separation of the *anima*:

ex vulva quoque feminis vehemens malum nascitur ... interdum etiam sic exanimat, ut tamquam comitiali morbo prosternat. distat tamen hic casus eo, quod neque oculi vertuntur nec spumae profluunt nec nervi distenduntur: sopor tantum est. *Med. 4.27*: 1A.

A violent disorder also originates from the uterus of women ... Occasionally it can even cause fainting (*exanimat*), in such a way that they are thrown to the ground like in an epileptic attack. It differs though from the latter, in that neither are the eyes turned, nor is there any foaming, nor spastic paralysis: such is the level of drowsiness.

---

[1] von Staden (2010: 13).

Note how fainting in this passage is distinguished from an epileptic seizure (another form of total loss of consciousness) and assimilated to *sopor* (drowsy impaired consciousness). Unlike Celsus' understanding of delirium, which presented – as discussed above – very clear boundaries with sleep, fainting was in its peripheries. This also becomes patent in the chapter on epilepsy (*morbus comitialis*), where the impossibility of *lethargic* patients waking up (*exper gisci*) contrasted with the spontaneous coming round (*ad se revertitur*)[2] of epileptic individuals. In other words, on two occasions the author explicitly discusses the difference between sleep and total loss of consciousness, which suggests that he perceived them as related or similar presentations.

It does make sense – from a purely clinical standpoint – that if sleep is an all-or-nothing phenomenon, with almost no intermediate states (as Celsus seems to have conceived it), sleep and fainting can be readily confused but not sleep and delirium. The idea seems perfectly reasonable when applying the anaesthetic model: in dreamless sleep (Celsus very seldom mentions dreams or parasomnia), as well as in drowsy states, alertness, connectedness and responsiveness are reduced. In the case of deep sleep – as in the total loss of consciousness – they are virtually abolished.

In summary, in agreement with Celsus' constant search for the 'middle way', there is a formal (mainly terminological) agreement with the Hippocratic forerunners and a coincidence in the notion of separation, but – as I will argue below – a rather different idea of the soul.

Aretaeus' take on this matter raises similar concerns:

ἔκλυσιν δὲ γουνάτων καὶ αἰσθήσιος πρόσκαιρον νάρκην καὶ ἀψυχίην καὶ κατάπτωσιν, λιποθυμίην καλέομεν. *SD I.7. CMG (H).III*: 44, 20–1.

The knees giving way, temporary numbness of perceptions, fainting (*apsuchiê*) and collapse is called 'swoon'(*lipothumiên*).

First of all, it is worthwhile to remark that one of the components of *lipothumiê* is *apsuchiê*, thereby distancing – from a terminological viewpoint – from the absolute synonymy found in the Hippocratic collection. In this passage, *apsuchiê* does not seem to encompass the

---

[2] *Med. 3.23*:1–2.

loss of perceptions (otherwise Aretaeus would not have needed to add them independently to the list). Additionally, this definition appears in the chapter devoted to paralysis, in which *lipothumiê* is framed as an extreme version of it. In other words, it is the total suppression of motor capacities and perceptions. As a result, the passage and the context in which it appears both suggest that movement and sensitivity were central components of swoons, and that they were both encompassed in the idea of *leipothumiê* but not in the notion of *apsuchiê*. The question still remains, though, whether Aretaeus was using these terms in a lexicalised manner or if he was implying some separation of the *psuchê* by using them.

The role of the *psuchê* in swoons is rather unclear, for most explanations involve humours (mainly blood), different forms of heat and tension. Aretaeus often discusses fainting in connection with excessive blood-letting,[3] and the role of the soul in them is erratic (to say the least). Only once does the *psuchê* appear as a relevant component where it separates from the body. It is in the treatment of *pleuritis*, where large phlebotomies are recommended:

... τὸ δὲ πλῆθος μὴ μέχρι λειποθυμίης· περιπνευμονίην γὰρ ἐπιφοιτῆσαι κίνδυνος, ἢν τὸ σῶμα ἐπιψυχθὲν τὴν ψυχὴν ἐκλείπῃ. εἴσω γὰρ τὰ ὑγρὰ ξυνθέει, τῆς ἐκτὸς ἀφαιρεθέντα θέρμης τε καὶ τάσιος. *CA I.10. CMG (H).V*: 114, 5–6.

... the amount [of blood withdrawn] should not be enough to cause a swoon, for this can add the risk of *pneumonia* if the chilled body releases the soul (*psuchê*). Indeed, the moisture accumulates inside, having been separated from the heat (*thermê*) and tension (*tasis*).

In this passage, Aretaeus relates the release of the *psuchê* in swoons to becoming cold after excessive loss of blood. Beyond the coincidence with Hippocratic (and Celsian) works, this example is quite illustrative of his lax eclecticism. Indeed, the particle *gar* seems to be suggesting that the soul – which can be either associated with heat (*thermê*) and tension (*tasis*), or only with tension if we interpret that the heat is exclusive to the blood – is being released along with the blood. We can point out, therefore, a faint family resemblance with two different traditions. On the one hand, blood was considered to be hot in humoural theories,

---

[3] This cause also makes sense to modern medicine: a large haemorrhage, or perhaps the mere sight of blood, can produce loss of consciousness.

hence its loss was equated with coldness. On the other, the assimilation of the *psuchê* with heat and tension reminds us of the *pneuma* as the key constituent of the soul, according to Stoic philosophy.[4] However, the blood is also moist in humoural theories (whereas the moisture stays in the body, according to this explanation), and there are no allusions to *pneuma* in this passage. Furthermore, the technical word that the Stoics frequently used to talk about tension was *tonos* rather than *tasis*.[5] Could Aretaeus be referring, instead, to the tone of the muscles, which is lost when one collapses? There is no explicit evidence of this either. Perhaps he is talking about yet another kind of tension: the tension presented in the chapter on *sunkopê* where the disease causes a 'weakening of the tension of nature'.[6] Undoubtedly, the concept of family resemblance (which characterises Aretaeus' eclecticism) describes this tangle of ideas quite accurately: we can see that his explanations have features in common with different traditions, but he is not strictly following any of them, because there are also important discrepancies.

Going back to the role of the *psuchê* in swoons, in most other descriptions, the soul is not mentioned. Such is the case with *melancholia*, which offers yet another example of Aretaeus' method:

... σμικρόν [αἷμα] ἀφαιρέειν, ὁκόσον αἴσθηται τομῆς ἡ δύναμις οὐκ ἐλεγχθείη δὲ ἐπὶ τῷ τόνῳ ... τόδε ἐστὶ τῆς φύσιος ὁ χῶρος καὶ ἡ τροφή. ἢν ὦν τοῦ δέοντος ἀφέλῃς, ἀτροφίη ἡ φύσις ἐξίσταται τῆς ἕδρης. *CD I.5. CMG (H).VII*: 156, 7–8, 10–11.

... a small amount [of blood] should be let; enough that the strength [of the patient] may perceive the incision, but not be tested as to its force ... [for] this [the blood] is the location and the nourishment of the *phusis*. Thus, if you let more than is necessary, the *phusis* will be expelled from its seat due to lack of nourishment.

---

[4] Shields (2018: 36).
[5] There are later testimonies that the terms (*tasis* and *tonos*) were used as synonyms:

ὁ δὲ ὡς τάσις τόνος λέγεται *Cleonides* (Musicus). *Introductio harmonica*: Sect. 12 line 38.
ἡ δὲ τάσις ἐλέχθη τόνος. *Theon* (Phil). *De utilitate mathematicae*: p. 70 line 12.
τόνος δέ ἐστιν ἡ τάσις τοῦ πνεύματος· *Commentaria in Dionysii Thracis Artem Grammaticam* Comm. et Gramm: Scholia Londinensia (partim excerpta ex Heliodoro). These examples were taken from *Thesaurus Linguae Graecae*® Digital Library. Ed. M. C. Pantelia. University of California, Irvine. http://www.tlg.uci.edu (last accessed 2 November 2019).
[6] ἔκλυσις τοῦ τόνου τῆς φύσιος, *SA II.3. CMG (H).II*: 23, 4.

Here it is the *phusis* and not the *psuchê* that seems to be expelled with the blood in large phlebotomies. Additionally, this *phusis* is associated – like the *psuchê* before – with tension (*tonos* in this case), carried in the blood and assimilated to food. The *tonos* might well be referring to the *phusis* (like in *sunkopê*) and may be a synonym of *tasis* from the previous example.[7] However, we can once again only talk about family resemblance and not adherence to Pneumatic thought, because according to the Stoics, perceptions were part of the Psychic and not the Natural capacities, each of which represented a different level within the *scala naturae*.[8] Also against this hypothesis is the equivalence between *psuchê* and *phusis*, which the analogy between the commented-on passages appears to be suggesting.[9]

Therefore, Aretaus' understanding of fainting presents echoes, resemblances and discrepancies with other theories (one of them being the separation of the soul). However, none of them is clearly predominant nor followed consistently. As a matter of fact, his lax eclectic method consisted of combining different elements of different theories at his convenience, regardless of possible contradictions or incoherence between them.

Sunkopê

I will begin the post-Hellenistic authors' approach to the second form of total loss of consciousness with the description of *sunkopê* that appears in the *Anonymus Parisinus*, because it offers a comprehensive exposition of certain elements that will partially reappear in Celsus, Aretaeus and other post-Hellenistic sources.

ὀνομαστὶ μὲν τοῦ πάθους οἱ παλαιοὶ οὐκ ἐμνήσθησαν ὡς καθ' αὑτὸ γινομένου, ἐπιγινομένου ... μάλιστα δὲ στομάχῳ, ὅ περ καλεῖται καρδία.[10] δι' ὅ περ τινὲς

---

[7] Especially considering that the strength is affected, which could be a way of referring to the muscular tone, that naturally disappears during swoons.

[8] Annas (1992: 71–2).   [9] Annas (1992: 51).

[10] The ambiguity of the terms *stomachos* and *kardias* has led to confusion from antiquity up to the present day. As Lonie (1981: 268–88) has remarked, some Hippocratic authors used *kardiôgmon* or *kardialgia* to refer to liver-related symptoms. Similarly, Galen commented on Thucydides' use of *kardia* to refer to the orifice of the stomach (*PHP. LCL II.8*, 2: 158, 17–30. *K.V*: 274–5). Such a discussion is also relevant in

Total loss of consciousness in post-Hellenistic authors

καρδίας ὑπέλαβον εἶναι τὸ πάθος ... γίνεσθαι δὲ αὐτὸ ... ἐκτονιζομένου τοῦ πνεύματος καὶ λυομένου ... τοῖς δὲ ὑπὸ συγκοπῶν ἁλοῦσι συνεδρεύει σφυγμὸς μικρός, συνδεδιωγμένος ... ἀναπνοὴ συνέχεται, καὶ ὡς ἂν ἐκλείποντες ἀντιλαμβάνονται τοῦ ἀέρος ... ἱδροῦσι δαψιλῶς τὰ ἄνω μέρη μάλιστα, ψυχρὸς δὲ αὐτοῖς ἐστιν ὁ ἱδρώς ... βάρος θώρακος συναισθαίνονται ... ἀποχωρίζουσι. *Anon. Paris. X.1, 1–2*: 72, 4–8; *X.2, 1–2*: 78, 14–21; *X.2, 3*: 74, 3.

The ancients have not mentioned this affection by name as a condition in its own right. It originates ... especially in the stomach, which is called *kardia*. Hence, some have assumed that it is an affection of the heart ... It occurs because the *pneuma* loses tension and dissolves ... The following symptoms accompany those suffering from *sunkopê*: small and fast pulse ... chaotic breathing, they hold the air as if they had fainted ... they sweat copiously, particularly in the upper parts. They have cold sweat ... feel heaviness in the chest ... [and] vomit.

As stated, there is no explicit mention in the Hippocratic collection of this disease (even if I have suggested above a feasible Hippocratic origin for it), and thus it is acknowledged by this author's remark that 'the ancients' did not give a name to this condition. Also, this – as well as most other ancient descriptions of *sunkopê*[11] – appears to be compatible with our current understanding of vasovagal syncopes (with hypopnea, cold sweat, gastrointestinal symptoms, cardiac symptoms and hypotension – hence the changes in the pulse). However, in this source it is not clear whether consciousness is actually lost. In most discussions about *sunkopê* there are usually hints that point towards some kind of impairment in the level of consciousness (in this case it is the breathing 'as if they had fainted'), but it is seldom explicit whether the patient actually passed out or not.

Lucretius' re-creation of the Athenian plague, where the poet translates the original Greek *kardia* (*Thuc.II. 49.3*) referring to the stomach, as *cor* (*Rer. nat.VI. 1152*) (see Commager 1957: 105–6). In modern languages this ambiguity has given rise to lay expressions such as 'heartburn' or '*mal du coeur*' to describe the symptoms triggered by gastro-esophagic reflux. As a matter of fact, the 'cardia' is nowadays the anatomical name of the distal orifice of the oesophagus (which is exactly the same as the proximal orifice of the stomach). In the case of *sunkopê* it is likely that *stomachos* refers to the epigastric region, in which symptoms that usually accompany vasovagal syncopes (such as local distress, nausea, vomiting) are perceived. It is not unlikely that this terminological and semantic ambiguity has generated the debate concerning the origin of the condition (the stomach versus the heart), which will be discussed below.
[11] For example, the Pseudo-Galenic *Introduction* (*CUF XIII.14*: 52, 23–8; 53,1–7) and the Pseudo-Galenic *Medical definitions 265* (*K.XIX.420*: 15–17; 421, 1–3).

168

Celsus' take on *cardiacum* matches the previous description quite closely. In his narrative, it is clearly differentiated from *defectio animae*, because the problem is in the body, specifically in the stomach:[12]

> id autem nihil aliud est quam nimia inbecillitas corporis, quod stomacho languente inmodico sudore digeritur. licetque protinus scire id esse, ubi venarum exigui inbecillique pulsus sunt … pedibus … et cruribus siccioribus atque frigentibus. *Med. 3.19*: 1.

It [*Cardiacum*] is nothing else than excessive weakness of the body, which is wasted away by excessive sweating because the stomach is weak. It can be immediately spotted when the pulse of the blood vessels is small and weak … feet and legs are drier [than the other sweaty parts of the body] and cold.

Then, later in the chapter devoted to this condition (*Med. 3.19*) he warns *si verendum est ne deficiat*… ('if it is feared that the patient might faint… ').[13] This clarification indicates that *anima deficere* can certainly occur simultaneously with *cardiacum*, but is an occasional and independent symptom.[14] In other words, Celsus' approach to this disease was eminently physical, and both clinically and theoretically different from other forms of swoons.

In Aretaeus' text, on the other hand, the boundaries between *sunkopê* and *leipothumiê* are more blurred. Accordingly, there is no clear definition as to whether this disease primarily affects the body or the soul. The author begins the discussion by justifying the two names that he uses to designate the disease: *sunkopê* in the book on signs and causes, and *kardiakos* in the chapter devoted to its treatment. The former is due to the suddenness and strength of its presentation, whereas the latter points towards the affected organ. Trivial as this might seem, such an introduction positions the author at the opposite end of the ongoing debate concerning the *locus*

---

[12] Several other post-Hellenistic texts place the damage in the stomach, amongst them, the above-mentioned *Anonymus Parisinus* (*X*), the Pseudo-Galenic *Introduction* (*CUF XIII.14*) and the Pseudo-Galenic *Medical definitions* (*K.XIX*: 265).

[13] *Med. 3.19*: 4.

[14] Interestingly, a Hippocratic description of cerebral sphacelus shares many coincidences with Celsus' *cardiacum*: ἢν σφακελίσῃ ὁ ἐγκέφαλος, ὀδύνη … ἐπὶ τὴν καρδίην φοιτᾷ· καὶ ἀψυχίη καὶ ἱδρώς, καὶ ἄπνοος τελέθει ('if the brain becomes sphacelous, pain migrates towards the *cardias*, the patients faints, sweats and stops breathing'. *Morb. II. LCL 5*: 176, 10–12). However the author of *On diseases II* uses *apsuchiê* to refer to this fainting.

affectus.[15] Aretaeus outspokenly rejects the esophagic/gastric hypothesis, and places the affection in the heart, thereby expanding on his views on this organ:

τί δὲ καρδίης ἄλλο καιριώτερον ἐς ζωὴν ἢ ἐς θάνατον; οὐδὲ τὴν συγκοπὴν ἄπιστον τῆς καρδίης νοῦσον ἔμμεναι, ἢ αὐτὴν σίνος τῆς ἐν αὐτέῃ τοῦ ζῆν δυνάμιος ... ἔστι γὰρ τὸ πάθος λύσις τῶν δεσμῶν τῆς εἰς ζωὴν δυνάμιος, ἀντίξουν τῇ συστάσει τοῦ ἀνθρώπου ἐόν ... ἔνθα καὶ ἡ ψυχὴ καὶ ἡ φύσις αὐτέης, εἰς ἣν καὶ τὸ πάθος ἢ τῶν τῇδε δυνάμεων. ἔστι δὲ ἡ τῆς νούσου ἰδέη ἔκλυσις τοῦ τόνου τῆς φύσιος ἐπ' αἰτίῃ ψύξει καὶ ὑγρότητι. *SA II.3. CMG (H).II*: 21, 30; 22, 1–5; 23, 2–5.

What is more decisive for life or death other than the heart? It makes sense to posit that *sunkopê* is a disease of the heart, or an injury of its capacities for living ... Indeed, the affliction – being inimical to the human constitution – is the release from the bonds that fetter the capacity to live ... In it [the heart] are the soul and its nature; hence, also against it [the heart] are the diseases of its capacities [of the soul]. The form of this disease is, namely, a weakening of the tension of nature due to coldness and moistness.

In order to understand the implications of this passage, it is useful to contrast it with Aretaeus' own understanding of total loss of consciousness. There is a striking terminological and conceptual coincidence between *leipothumiê* and *sunkopê* in the treatise: the intervening faculties are the same, particularly the living-capacity (*eis zôên dunamios*); the *psuchê* and the *phusis* participate in both; the tension (*tonos*) has a similar role;[16] and the qualities cold and moist are as involved in *sunkopê* as they are in swoons (where heat is expelled during excessive phlebotomies, and humidity accumulates in the body once it releases the *psuchê*, *CA I.10. CMG (H).V*: 114, 5–6).

On the contrary, the importance of the blood has been overtaken in this passage by the heart. While blood seemed to be the seat of the *psuchê* and *phusis* in the passages on *leipopsuchiê*, in this description the heart plays that role. So far, therefore, we are

---

[15] The dispute is also mentioned by the author of the *Introduction* (*CUF XIII.14*: 52, 22–6), who seems to agree with the esophagic affection during *sunkopê* (like Celsus and the author of the *Anonymus Parisinus*).

[16] In another example of family resemblance regarding mechanisms, Aretaeus talked about the loss of tension in the *phusis* (ἔκλυσις τοῦ τόνου τῆς φύσιος, *SA II.3. CMG (H).II*: 23, 4), whereas the author of the *Anonymus Parisinus* referred to the loss of tension in the *pneuma* (ἐκτονιζομένου τοῦ πνεύματος καὶ λυομένου, *Anon. Paris. X.2, 1–2*: 78, 14–21).

170

presented with a condition that has many features in common with swoons concerning mechanisms and capacities affected, but a different location.

When looking at the symptoms the picture slightly changes:

σφυγμοὺς μικρούς, ἀδρανέας, πάταγον τῆς καρδίης, ἐπὶ πηδήσι καρτερῇ, σκοτόδινος, λειποθυμίη, νάρκη, καὶ παρέσιες μελέων, ἱδρὼς ἄσχετος, πουλύς, ψύξις ὅλου, ἀναισθησίη, ἀφωνίη. *SA II.3. CMG (H).II:* 22, 22–4.

Small and weak pulse, a loud heartbeat among strong palpitations, dizziness, swoon, numbness and weakness in the limbs, profuse uncontrollable sweating, coldness all over, insensitivity, speechlessness.[17]

The description of physical signs is much more thorough than in swoons, where the clinical presentation is barely mentioned. It is at this point that lax eclecticism comes into play because Aretaeus presents pathophysiological similarities with his own idea of fainting, but a clinical description that matches the presentation of *sunkopê* in the other post-Hellenistic treatises. In this sense, I partially disagree with Pigeaud's view that we cannot find in Aretaeus' work the type of careful observation that characterised the Hippocratic *Epidemics*, because the patient and his ailment become lost when forced into classification.[18] In fact, his work could be regarded as halfway between the exclusively patient-centred Hippocratic descriptions and other heavily theory-laden post-Hellenistic works. As this approach to *kardiakos* reveals, Aretaeus draws a lot from his own experience and is quite detailed in his clinical descriptions. Unlike his contemporaries, he clearly found important coincidences in the presentations of both conditions (swoons and *sunkopê*), along with their differences.[19]

In other words, Aretaeus conceived of two ways of losing consciousness: a simple one without accompanying symptoms

---

[17] Even to our contemporary understanding, this description seems like an eclectic amalgamation of the different types of syncopes that we nowadays distinguish.

[18] Pigeaud (1987: 81). Such a statement could certainly be argued about Celsus' and the other post-Hellenistic encyclopaedic endeavours (for example, the *Introduction*, the *Definitions* and the *Anonymus Parisinus*), but not about Aretaeus.

[19] Indeed, most of the other symptoms are equivalent. When comparing this passage with those where swoons are characterised, one finds *apsuchiê* in swoons and *leipothumiê* in *sunkopê*; ἔκλυσιν δὲ γουνάτων in fainting is the same as νάρκη, καὶ παρέσιες μελέων in *kardiakos*; and finally, αἰσθήσιος πρόσκαιρον νάρκην and ἀναισθησίη are virtually synonyms.

(often triggered by excessive blood-letting) and a more complex one (with bradycardia, hypotension and sweating) which constituted a disease in its own right, namely *sunkopê*.[20] This lax eclectic approach, therefore, enables Aretaeus to never disregard his own observations and allows him to subtly distance himself from the predominant understanding of the affection, where *leipothumiê* and *kardiakos* were completely unrelated conditions. He does not need to fit any finding within a fixed broader theoretical framework, because he can always find a convenient model to explain unexpected, unusual or unforeseen phenomena. In this way, the lack of a strict adherence to any sect provides him with the freedom to always come up with a suitable theoretical justification for whichever clinical manifestation he encounters.[21] Naturally, such justifications are often suggestive of a certain system of thought, but they never completely fit within any single and distinct one.[22] Thus, without an important amount of non-textual assumptions, we can only speculate which authors were informing which explanations.

Total loss of consciousness and ideas of the soul emerging in post-Hellenistic authors

In post-Hellenistic authors both the tension between body and soul, as well as the idea of a life-giving power within *psuchê/ anima*, are perhaps less emphatically stated (although still present) and strongly influenced by their methodological approach. Thus,

---

[20] The treatment of *phrenitis* offers further hints of an identity between swoons and *kardiakos*: in *phrenitis* excessive blood-letting can lead to a *sunkopê* (not to *leipothumiê*): ἀτὰρ καὶ φλέβα τάμνων μὴ πολλὸν ἀφαιρέειν ... φρενῖτις γὰρ εὔτρεπτον ἐς συγκοπὴν κακόν ('when cutting a vein not too much [blood] should be withdrawn ... for *phrenitis* is an evil that can easily turn into a *sunkopê*), *CA I.1. CMG (H).V*: 92, 21–2.

[21] Hence, he can say that the *psuchê* and the *phusis* depend on the blood, to justify fainting due to excessive blood-letting; then he can place them in the heart to explain *sunkopê*; and finally he can say that drawing too much blood can trigger a disease of the heart (in *phrenitis*).

[22] As discussed, debates on the location of the soul in the blood or the heart were present in the Hippocratic collection, and they might be underpinning these seemingly contradictory explanations. Moreover, as Thumiger (2017: 267) points out, the blood as the seat of emotions and cognition predates medical theorisations; and the blood around the heart as the location of *noêma* is Empedoclean ... all these traditions bear family resemblances with Aretaeus' assertions.

Celsus, as an encyclopaedist in search of the 'middle way', compiled different sources – including several Hippocratic ideas, which he tweaked in order to make them compatible with later philosophical theories – and transferred that knowledge into Latin. Aretaeus' lax eclecticism, on the other hand, allowed him to pick and choose more freely the elements that he needed from the various theories available to him.

Celsus: mens, animus *and* anima

Celsus offered no explicit philosophical speculation about the nature of certain constructs that he considered to be compromised in his descriptions of impaired consciousness. He gives no clear definition of the scope of the *mens*, the *animus* and the *anima*. As a result, his ideas about these matters can only be deduced from the way in which he used the terms, as well as how he explained the intervention of these concepts in his descriptions. So far, during the discussion on total loss of consciousness, I have mainly focused on the Hippocratic influence over Celsus in terms of vocabulary and his understanding of fainting as a separation of the soul.

Let us now revisit the above-quoted passage on *kephalaia*-associated total loss of consciousness and focus on an aspect that has remained undiscussed: the idea of the soul that emerges from it.[23]

The text illustrates how motion, vision, involuntary symptoms (such as vomiting), delirium (*mentis alienatio*) and speech are all independent of the soul (*anima*), because they are lost due to the disease before fainting actually occurs, namely, before the soul separates (*anima deficit*). Such a distinction suggests that many capacities that belonged to the Hippocratic *psuchê* – particularly the *mens* (the rational part affected by *vanas imagines* in *phrenesis*) – are no longer subsumed in the Celsian *anima*; on the contrary, they are independent of it. This presentation, therefore, hints at a different way of understanding and grouping ideas about

---

[23] To facilitate the readability of the analysis, I repeat here an excerpt from it that is relevant for my argument: *horror calidus, nervorum resolutio, oculorum caligo, mentis alienatio, vomitus sic ut vox supprimatur, vel sanguinis ex naribus cursus, sic ut corpus frigescat, anima deficiat* (*Med.* 4.2: 2).

perception, cognition and movement, as compared to the Hippocratic predecessors, and questions the equivalence between the Hippocratic *psuchê* and the Celsian *anima*.

From the various alternative models of the soul available to Celsus, I consider that his choice leaned towards a view that shared Asclepiadean or Epicurean elements. In order to pursue this idea further, it is necessary to provide some context; namely, to outline some ongoing philosophical debates.

Polito, following some simplification by Galen, has drawn attention to a bipolar division of philosophical thought at the time.[24] On the one hand, there were the philosophers of the 'mainstream tradition', who – broadly speaking – considered matter as a continuum and a unity and believed in intentionality and rationality, both in nature and in human beings (namely, a teleological stance). On the other hand, a group that included Asclepiades and Epicurus advocated – with certain nuances – a mechanistic view of the cosmos, which was formed of particles and void. Despite Vallance's reluctance to associate Asclepiades with Epicurus,[25] more recent scholarship has made a strong case for the important influence of Epicurean thought on Asclepiades' theories. Through different approaches, Leith[26] and Polito[27] agree that although there are some discrepancies, Asclepiades' debt to Epicurus is considerable, both at the physical level and in his psychology. As we shall see, in his approach to impaired consciousness Celsus negotiated various positions within contemporary philosophical debates, whilst at the same time trying to make these ideas compatible with the Hippocratic texts. Considering his frequent citations of Asclepiades,[28] it should not surprise us to see Celsus' narrative leaning towards the Asclepiadean/Epicurean side of the debate, even when trying to stick to the middle way.

In terms of vocabulary, several scattered allusions to psychological concepts remind us of Lucretius' Epicurean use of terminology, especially the interchangeability between *mens*, *animus* and

---

[24] Polito (2006: 288–93).   [25] Vallance (1990: 697–700).   [26] Leith (2009: 283–320).
[27] Polito (2006: 285–335).
[28] As Gautherie (2017: 52–3) accurately points out, Asclepiades is the only author in *On medicine* whose works ('On the preservation of health' and 'On common remedies') are explicitly mentioned.

consilium, which I have previously mentioned in the description of the third type of *insania* (*Men. III.18*: 19, 21). Such a synonymy also appears in *De rerum natura*, where the poet refers to '*consilium*, which we designate as *animus* and *mens*'.[29] This finding is rather eloquent, because several more or less contemporary examples testify that this correspondence was not universally accepted in Latin.[30]

Beyond the terminological coincidence, there seems to be a common theoretical background shared by *On medicine* and Lucretius' *On nature*, totally alien to the Hippocratic corpus. It consists of the primacy of the *mens* and *animus* over the *anima*. The followers of Epicurus had considered the soul to be comprised of a rational part located in the chest (*animus*) and a non-rational part diffused throughout the body (*anima*).[31] Lucretius is quite explicit about it: he considers the *animus* to be in control of the *anima* and through it, of the body.[32]

... facile ut quiuis hinc noscere possit
esse animam cum animo coniunctam, quae cum animi ui
percussast, exim corpus propellit et icit. *Rer. Nat. III*: 136–7.

... From this, anyone could easily realise that *anima* is united with *animus*, and that when it is shaken by the *animus*, it then moves and pushes the body.

Similarly, Celsus presents a causal link between *mens* and *anima*:

denique omnis calor iecur et lienem inflat, mentem hebetat; ut anima deficiat, ut sanguis prorumpat, efficit. *Med. 2.1*: 11.

---

[29] *consilium, quod nos animum mentemque uocamus* (*Rer. nat. LCL III*: 139).

[30] When talking about individuals out of control (*exisse ex potestate*), Cicero states that *non sunt in potestate mentis, cui regnum totius animi a natura tributum est* ('they are not under the control of their *mens*, which rules by nature over the *animus*', *TD LCL III*.5, 2: 236, 11–13). Similarly, Valerius Maximus utilises the terms with different connotations. He uses *animus* to talk about character traits such as bravery (*Dicta et facta memorabilia III. 2.5*: 238, 22), endurance (*III.3 ext. 1*: 274, 16), etc. Also, he clearly distinguishes *animus* from *mens* when he states: *transgrediar ad saluberrimam partem animi, moderationem, quae mentes nostras impotentiae et temeritatis incursu transversas ferri non patitur* ('I shall pass to the most advantageous aspect of the character (*animus*), moderation, which prevents our minds (*mens*) from being carried away by an impulse of helplessness and indiscretion', *Dicta et facta memorabilia IV. praef*: 336, 1–2).

[31] Verde (2020: 89–119) convincingly argues that the division between a rational and a non-rational part of the soul was a key feature of several Epicurean followers, and possibly an idea developed by Epicurus himself.

[32] Bailey (1947: 1011).

Finally, heat produces inflammation in the liver and the spleen, and weakens the
mens so that the patient faints (*anima deficiat*).

This excerpt illustrates the thorough work carried out by Celsus in
order to achieve his middle way. Hippocratic doctors had certainly
made a related claim in the *Aphorisms*, although they had not ventured
any causation: τὸ θερμὸν βλάπτει ταῦτα ... γνώμης νάρκωσιν ...
λειποθυμίας... ('heat produces the following damages ... benumbing
of the *gnômê* ... fainting spells ... ').[33] Celsus, while apparently
translating these ideas into Latin, is actually tweaking his sources and
adding a heavy Epicurean bias to them, which, furthermore, was
opposed to the Hippocratic texts, where *phronêsis*, *gnômê*, *sunesis*
and *nous* were subordinated to the *psuchê*. In this way – through the *ut*
final clause – Celsus subordinated the alleged equivalent of the latter
(the *anima*) to the former (*mens/animus*).

In a similar manner, we can find coincidences in the implications of such ideas. In *On nature* it is stated *hic exsultat ... pauor
ac metus ... hic ergo mens animusquest* ('here [in the chest] we
feel terror ... and fear ... hence, here are the *mens* and the
animus').[34] Celsus avoids the theoretical explanation and the
localisation in the body, but maintains the consequences of such
an understanding, namely, the involuntary automatic bodily reactions associated with the *psuchê* in the Hippocratic collection such
as teeth being on edge, fear, anger and pulse changes (*Hum. CMG*
9: 18, 3–13), which are caused in *On medicine* by the *mens* and the
animus instead of the *anima*: *is, qui menti suae non est ... dentibus
stridet* ('those whose *mens* is not sound ... grind their teeth');[35]
*eas [venas] concitare solet ... metus et ira et quilibet alius animi
adfectus* ('fear, anger and any other affection of the *animus* usually
excites [the pulse]').[36] Although the terms used by Celsus could
suggest a Hippocratic mark to them, the idea underpinning the
roles that he attributes to *animus* and *anima* appear to be rather
Epicurean. Once again his translation is not innocent.

Another aspect that can be explained by Celsus' adherence to this
Epicurean-informed functional division of the *anima* into a rational
and non-rational part is the way in which he conceived the relationship

---

[33] *Aph. LCL* 5.16: 160, 15–17.   [34] *Rer. nat. LCL III*: 141–2.   [35] *Med.* 2.6: 5.
[36] *Med.* 3.6: 6.

between the different presentations of impaired consciousness, particularly the drowsy one. I have mentioned in Part II of this book that unlike many predecessors and contemporaries, Celsus' take on sleep avoided discussing HOFs, philosophical or physiological aspects.[37] Notably, *On medicine* did not mention intermediate states between wakefulness and sleep, but posited an utter separation between them, which strongly contrasted with the fuzzy edges that it did suggest between sleep and total loss of consciousness.

The Epicurean notion of the *anima* partially – not completely – expelled from the body during sleep (explicit in Lucretius)[38] can justify these fuzzy edges, for this idea is not far from Celsus' notion of a swoon (*anima deficere*). In this way, an *anima* partially expelled during drowsy impaired consciousness and more fully expelled during total loss of consciousness would provide a sound theoretical explanation for the blurred boundaries between these two presentations. Furthermore, the idea of a complete lack of connectedness during sleep (even from one's own perceptions)[39] would also be consistent with this idea of partial separation of the *anima*. As a matter of fact, it is the *anima* diffused throughout the body where perceptions belong, according to Epicurus' followers.[40] In other words, the union between body and soul, which allowed sentience,[41] would be interrupted during sleep because of the partial separation of the *anima*.[42]

Additionally, this model also explains the complete separation that Celsus suggested between delirium and sleep. In wakeful impaired consciousness it was not the *anima*, but the *mens* and

[37] In the Hippocratic corpus sleep had been related to the *psuchê*, the *gnômê* and *phronêsis*. Similar associations persisted in the post-Hellenistic tradition. Thus, the Pseudo-Galenic *Definitions* considers sleep as ἄνεσις ψυχῆς κατὰ φύσιν ἀπὸ τῶν περάτων ἐπὶ τὸ ἡγεμονικόν ('the natural loosening of the *psuchê* from the periphery towards the *hêgemonikon*', *Def. Med. 127. K.XIX*: 381, 14–15).

[38] *cum sopor ... tum nobis animam ... esse putandumst eiectamque foras; non omnem* ('during slumber ... our *anima* is thought to be expelled out [of the body], not completely', *Rer. nat. LCL 4*: 921–3).

[39] I have highlighted above how Celsus conceived sleep as a process during which the individual is radically disconnected from his surroundings to the extent that he cannot even perceive his own pain.

[40] Annas (1992: 144).   [41] Verde (2020: 93).

[42] In this regard, Dossey (2013: 226–7) also associated certain ideas akin to a near-separation or extreme disconnection between body and soul during sleep (which left the body virtually devoid of the capacities provided by the soul) with Latin late antiquity. Strobl (2002: 36) and Stock (2010: 105) support this idea.

the *animus*, that became affected. The independence of sleep from the *mens* seems to be hinted at by the above-quoted definitions of *lethargy* and *phrenitis* (as remarked, *mens* is mentioned in the explanation of the latter but not of the former).[43] The lack of a link between sleeping and the *animus* is also present:

ante adversam autem valetudinem . . . quaedam notae oriuntur, quarum omnium commune est aliter se corpus habere atque consuevit . . . si gravior somnus pressit, si tumultuosa somnia fuerunt, si saepius expergiscitur aliquis quam adsuevit deinde iterum soporatur; si corpus dormientis circa partes aliquas contra consuetudinem insudat . . . item si marcet animus. . . *Med. 2.2*: 1; 2–3.

But prior to poor health . . . certain signs appear, all of which share in common that the body becomes different from its usual state: . . . if heavier sleep oppresses, if there are turbulent dreams, if the patient wakes up more often than usual and then falls back into sleep; if the sleeping body sweats around certain parts that it usually does not . . . Similarly, if the *animus* languishes. . .

This passage makes a clear distinction between types of symptoms that announce poor health. Among them, there are, on the one hand, sleep-related disturbances and, on the other, affections of the *animus*. They are both similarly predictive of illnesses; however, they are presented as completely independent from one another.

Finally, as suggested by some Hippocratic doctors and by Epicurus himself,[44] Celsus considered the soul to separate with death. In the *prooemium* (42), '*animam amittere*' designates death as a result of vivisection, thereby suggesting that by cutting the body the *anima* is lost.[45] An indirect hint of the close relationship between the separation caused by death and that caused by a swoon can be found in the terminology chosen in the pharmacological section. When discussing wounds in internal organs, Celsus recommends wine for those *ex profluvio sanguinis intermorientes* ('fainting (*intermorientes*) of haemorrhage').[46] The idea of dying

---

[43] In eo [phrenesis] *difficilior somnus, prompta ad omnem audaciam mens est: in hoc* [lethargo] *marcor et inexpugnabilis paene dormiendi necessitas* ('whereas in it [*phrenesis*] sleeping is difficult, and the *mens* is prone to any kind of insolence; in *lethargy* there is torpor and an almost overpowering need of sleep', *Med. 3.20*: 1).

[44] τοῦτο δὲ πᾶν αἱ δυνάμεις τῆς ψυχῆς δηλοῦσι καὶ τὰ πάθη καὶ αἱ εὐκινησίαι καὶ αἱ διανοήσεις καὶ ὧν στερόμενοι θνῄσκομεν ('The capacities of the soul, its affections, its ease of motion, its thoughts, and its features whose loss causes our death demonstrate all this', *Ep. Hdt. 63*: 2).

[45] Quite close to the Hippocratic τὴν ψυχὴν ἀφῆκε (*Int. LCL 39*: 176, 3 and *Int. LCL 40*: 178, 13–14).

[46] *Med. 5.26*: 25B.

(*morior*) is implicit in the term. There is a similar occurrence in the Hippocratic *Epidemics V*, where not only the resemblance of the condition, but also the verb chosen (*ekthnêskô*) refers to death: ἐξέθανε πεντάκις ὡς τεθνάναι δοκεῖν ('she fainted five times, she even seemed to be dead').[47] Once again, it might look as though the encyclopaedist was strictly following his Hippocratic predecessors; however, there is also an Epicurean explanation underpinning the choice of terms. Beyond the separation of the soul, the choice of *anima* and not *animus* or *mens* suggests an Epicurean influence. As Annas has accurately remarked, unlike the Stoics, who talked about the *hêgemonikon* (the ruling part) to refer to the soul as a whole, Lucretius uses *anima* (the non-rational part) for the same purpose,[48] as Celsus also seems to be doing.

Aretaeus: an erratic role of the soul in his eclectic approach to fainting

I have already pointed out the difficulty in defining a distinct notion of the soul in Aretaeus' work. Accordingly, despite the fact that in this condition patients collapse, loose movement, sensitivity and cognition, the author conveys neither a clear nor a consistent association between body and soul, and presents important contradictions regarding the way in which the mental capacities relate to the notion of the *psuchê*. Once again, Aretaeus seems to be combining different theories that partially overlap and partially disagree with each other.

In terms of the body–soul tension, both types of loss of consciousness (*leipothumiê*[49] and *sunkopê/kardiakos*)[50] suggest a separation of the *psuchê* from the body, but – as stated – the notion is rather erratic. Not only because the author uses *psuchê* and *phusis* interchangeably in swoons, whereas nature (*phusis auteês*) seems to be subordinated to the soul (*psuchê*) in *sunkopê*, but also because in the former condition he implies that the *psuchê* is located in the blood, whereas in the latter its seat is the heart. (I have already mentioned how Aretaeus had distanced himself from the seemingly mainstream conception of *sunkopê* by

---

[47] *Epid. V. CUF 42, 1*: 21, 4–5.   [48] Annas (1992: 145).
[49] *CA I.10. CMG (H).V*: 114, 5 and *CD I.5. CMG (H).VII*: 156, 10.
[50] *SA II.3. CMG (H).II*: 21, 30; 22, 1–5; 23, 2–3.

choosing a different *locus affectus* – the heart instead of the stomach[51] – and by involving the *psuchê* and not merely the body.) The role of the *psuchê* as a life force is explicitly mentioned as 'the capacity to live' in *sunkopê* (*eis zôên dunamios*). An idea akin to a life force is considered to be lost in *leipothumiê*-causing phlebotomies during the treatment of *apoplexy*: τὸ σμικρὸν αἷμα δυνατώτατον, καὶ [ἡ] ἀλέη τῆς ζωῆς τοῦ σκήνεος καὶ τῆς τροφῆς ἐόν ('even a little blood is most powerful, for it is the heat of the life of the body and of nourishment').[52] However, it is not clear whether this ἀλέη τῆς ζωῆς τοῦ σκήνεος καὶ τῆς τροφῆς is equivalent to the other form of heat (*thermê*), or in any way associated with tension (*tasis*, *tonos*), with the soul (*psuchê*) or with nature (*phusis*), all of which Aretaeus had also involved in *leipothumiê* caused by excessive blood-letting. In any case, it sounds intuitively coherent that this author conceived total loss of consciousness at the very boundary between life and death, if he understood that the heat of life was lost during swoons, as was the capacity to live during *sunkopê*. He seems to be suggesting that the loss of the *psuchê* or the *phusis* or their tension in the form of heat left an inert and cold body (not too different from a corpse).

Concerning the relationship between mental capacities and the notion of the *psuchê*, in the discussion on HOFs I briefly mentioned some contradictions. As opposed to his usual opposition *aisthêsis–gnômê*, Aretaeus opposed, in the *prooemium* to the books on chronic illnesses, *aisthêsis* to *psuchê*.[53] Moreover, in his discussions on *leipothumiê* and *sunkopê* the *psuchê* is involved, but there is no mention of the *gnômê*. Could this be suggesting, perhaps, that he was symphoretically thinking of them in these passages as related notions (especially considering that the *gnômê* also tended to be anatomically located in the heart)?

Although this hypothesis is plausible given Aretaeus' lax eclecticism, there are passages that contradict such an identity. A rather

---

[51] In this respect, there are further examples of syncretism: in the chapter on treatment, Aretaeus suggests that the condition can alternatively be caused by φλεγμασίη τις ὑποχονδρίου, ἢ ἥπατος ('certain inflammation of the hypochondria and the liver', *CA II.3. CMG (H).VI*: 126, 22–3).

[52] *CA I.4. CMG (H).V*: 103, 1–2.

[53] ἀλλ' ἐς πολλὰ τὴν αἰσθησίην ἐκτρέπει, ἀλλὰ καὶ τὴν ψυχὴν ἐκμαίνει (*SD I.1. CMG (H).III*: 36, 16–17).

puzzling phenomenon described during *sunkopê* – unheard of in the other sources – suggests a differentiation between *psuchê* and *gnômê*:

ἐπὶ δὲ τοῖσι καρδιώσσουσι καὶ αἴσθησις ὀξύτεροι, ὡς ἰδεῖν καὶ ἀκοῦσαι μᾶλλον ἢ πρόσθεν, καὶ γνώμη εὐσταθέστεροι, καὶ ψυχῇ καθαρώτεροι, καὶ τάδε οὐκ εἰς τὰ παρεόντα μοῦνον, καὶ ἐς τὰ μέλλοντα μάντιες ἀτρεκέες. *SA II. CMG (H).II*: 22, 26– 8; 23, 1.

Amongst those who suffer from the heart, perceptions are sharper, so that they can see and hear better than before, their *gnômê* is clearer, their soul (*psuchê*) is purer and not only can they accurately prophesy about the present, but also about the future.

Beyond the inconsistencies with the other clinical features presented in the rest of the chapter, this situation of clairvoyance offers a division of the sphere of consciousness into three components, namely, *aisthêsis*, *gnômê* and *psuchê* (in the similar passage with prophetic visions caused by *kausôn*, the tripartite division included *aisthêsis*, *gnômê* and *dianoia*).[54]

It appears that in an extreme version of Aretaeus' lax eclectic approach, the idea of the *psuchê* that emerges from the analysis of total loss of consciousness is syncretic (in particular, the interplay between *psuchê* and *phusis* illuminates how some passages suggest a family resemblance with Stoic philosophy, whereas others contradict it). Like most of the other concepts and numerous theories within his reach (considering that he was a learned physician), Aretaeus used the soul variously in different contexts, which allowed him to explain certain findings. On most occasions though (*psuchê* is a relatively infrequent term), he disregarded the notion altogether and used alternative constructs to provide a theoretical correlate of his apparently vast practical experience.

Finally, in line with Aretaeus' ill-defined *psuchê*, the connection between the different forms of impaired consciousness does not

---

[54] The three concepts seem to be at the same level, which disproves Pigeaud's hypothesis that Aretaeus considers '*sensation et pensée*' (*aisthêsis* and *gnômê*) as two manifestations of the *psuchê* (Pigeaud 1987: 91). Actually, I do not think that we can talk about a *théorie de la connaissance* in Aretaeus, as this scholar suggests. Aretaeus certainly does often oppose these two notions, but – as I have pointed out, mainly to distinguish mental illness from impaired consciousness – on other occasions he contrasts them with other concepts.

point directly towards the soul itself. However, the three prototypical presentations do evoke elements that were vaguely associated with the soul, such as heat, tension and *pneuma*.[55] These are the main components often related to the soul that – in one way or another – tend to be present in most discussions on conditions involving impaired consciousness.

---

[55] A benumbed (*nenarkômenon*) *pneuma* can cause fainting due to lack of *tonos* (*CA I. CMG (H).V.1*: 97, 25).

CHAPTER 15

GALEN'S TWO WAYS OF LOSING CONSCIOUSNESS

In the previous chapters I have highlighted the consistency of Galen's system in tackling diseases. With all the other forms of impaired consciousness he felt quite comfortable discussing specific imbalances of qualities in determined locations, whether by primary affection or sympathy. With total loss of consciousness this partially changes: as with his predecessors, we can single out in his work two different forms, but one of them – *leipopsuchiê* – offers a breach in his otherwise consistent systematisation. The complete shutdown that occurs during swoons challenges his extremely compartmentalised and rational theoretical framework. As a matter of fact, it is not as frequently referred to as it was in the previous authors, and it is less clearly explained than any other type of alteration of consciousness. *Sunkopê*, on the other hand, fits better in this comprehensive model and is more widely discussed throughout his work.

Fainting/*leipothumiê*

The terminology for swoons seems rather standardised. Like in the Hippocratic corpus, words are used interchangeably and convey an idea of separation and withdrawal: *leipothumiê*, *leipopsuchiê*, *ekluomai* and *ekleipô*. However, neither the role of the soul nor its release from the body are explicitly mentioned, particularly because his approach to the *locus affectus* in this condition is erratic. Despite the loss of all possible cognitive functions, fainting is related to different *archai*, and not only the brain – the seat of his *hêgemonikon* – as one would expect if swoons were construed as a psychic condition:

ὑποφεύγει γὰρ κἂν τούτοις ἐπὶ τὴν ἀρχὴν ἡ ἔμφυτος θερμασία λυομένη θ' ἅμα καὶ κατασβεννυμένη. ὅπου δὲ θάνατον ἐπιφέρει τὰ τοιαῦτα τῶν παθῶν, οὐδὲν δήπου θαυμαστὸν εἰ καὶ λειποψυχίαν. *Caus. Symp. II.5. K.VII*: 194, 8–11.

The innate heat released and quenched withdraws from them [patients in pain] towards its principle (*archê*). Where these affections bring about death, it is not surprising if they also cause swoons.

We can recognise some well-known elements associated with *leipopsuchiê*, namely the loss of heat and the idea of a near-death experience. The *archê* referred to is the heart, which carries the innate heat according to Galen's system (*UP 6.7 [III.436 K.]*). This is – with some reservations – in agreement with a passage of *On the affected parts*, where he mentions *ekluomenoi* patients while discussing heart conditions:

ὁ θάνατος ἕπεται κατὰ δὲ τὰς ὀργανικὰς ἐξαιφνίδιος, ἀλλ᾽ ἐπὶ προηγουμένοις σημείοις, ὧν ἕν μέν ἐστι καὶ τὸ πρὸς Ἱπποκράτους εἰρημένον, οἷον οἱ ἐκλυόμενοι πολλάκις καὶ ἰσχυρῶς ἄνευ φανερῆς προφάσεως, ἐξαπίνης τελευτῶσιν. *Loc. Aff.* 5.2. *K.VIII*: 303, 4–8.

[In large *duskrasias*] sudden death occurs when they affect the organs, but only subsequent to some predisposing symptoms, one of which was mentioned by Hippocrates: 'those who faint (*ekluomenoi*) often and severely without an evident reason die suddenly'.

Because he was tackling diseases of the heart, it is reasonable to think that he is referring to that organ; however, he uses a plural (*kata tas organikas*), which leaves the matter rather vague. On the other hand, in *On the doctrines of Hippocrates and Plato*, after explaining that the soul dwells in the body of the brain, and that the *pneuma* is its primary instrument for perception and motion, he states:

κενωθέντος αὐτοῦ κατὰ τὰς τρώσεις αὐτίκα μὲν οἷόν περ νεκρὸν γίγνεσθαι τὸ ζῷον, ἀθροισθέντος δὲ αὖθις ἀναβιώσκεσθαι. *PHP. LCL VII.3*: 446, 13–15. *K.V*: 606.

Once [*the pneuma*] is depleted through wounds, the animal immediately becomes like a corpse; when collected again, it revives.

Although there is no explicit mention of a swoon, Galen is – in all likelihood – describing a fainting patient, and he construes such fainting as a near-death experience. Of note is the fact that contrary to the previous passage, the phenomenon seems to be located in the brain and the main lost component is *pneuma*.

Finally, excessive blood-letting can also cause fainting: ἀφαιρῶ τοίνυν αὐτοῦ τοσοῦτον ἐξεπίτηδες ὡς λειποθυμίαν ἐπιγενέσθαι ('I deliberately took from him enough [blood] to bring about swooning (*leipothumiê*)').[1] The cooling effect of phlebotomies makes them the treatment of choice against continuous fevers, for εἰς ἐναντίαν κατάστασιν ἀφικνεῖται τάχιστα ψυχόμενον ἐν τῇ λειποθυμίᾳ τὸ σῶμα ('the body cooled during a swoon (*leipothumiê*) reaches the opposite state [to the heat of fever] very quickly').[2] However, the reason why such a bleeding causes fainting appears to be related to nourishment:

οὗτοί γε φέρουσιν, ἀλλὰ τὰς καλουμένας λειποψυχίας· ἐκλύονται γὰρ, εἰ μὴ τρέφοιντο συνεχέστερον οἱ τοιοῦτοι. *MM XII.5. LCL III*: 274, 19–20. *K.X*: 845.

These [unconcocted humours can] bring about swooning (*leipopsuchia*). These patients faint (*ekluontai*) if they are not constantly nourished.[3]

If we consider that food is turned into blood in order to be delivered throughout the body and nourish it, it is not surprising that the excessive loss of blood can be equated with insufficient or ineffective nourishment (uncooked humours do not feed the patients). However, in Galen's system nourishment and the production of blood were related to the desiderative soul, and hence to the liver.

In summary, there is no single coherent explanation of *leipothumiê* in Galen's work. He seems to be trying to make clinical findings (such as loss of heat, loss of blood and near-death experience) compatible with his system, where conditions could be addressed by determining a *locus affectus* and a specific *duskrasia* that disturbed it. Different combinations of those elements are certainly present; however, there is no consistency to them. Although the heart seems to have some pre-eminence, in different treatises a different part of his three-part *psuchê* seems to be involved. Possibly, the difficulty of linking this kind of fainting to the rational soul stems from Galen's adherence to his all-encompassing model. The actual experience of fainting as a consequence of blood-letting must have made it difficult for him to associate the phenomenon with the *hêgemonikon* (despite the loss of all cognitive capacities): the blood was related to the heart and the arteries according to his physiology and not to the brain, which used *pneuma*.[4] As a result, it would have been difficult for him to justify

[1] *MM IX. 4. LCL III*: 468, 14. *K.X*: 612.   [2] *MM IX.4. LCL III*: 468, 17–18. *K.X*: 612.
[3] Note the synonymy between *leipopsuchia* and *ekluomai*.
[4] πρῶτον ὄργανον ὑπάρχον τῇ ψυχῇ πρὸς τὸ διαπέμπειν εἰς ἅπαντα τὰ μέρη τοῦ σώματος αἴσθησίν τε καὶ κίνησιν ('the main tool contained in the *psuchê* to send perception and movement to all the parts of the body', *Loc. Aff. 4.3. K.VIII*: 233, 4–6).

that losing blood affected the mind without undermining his own physiological understanding.

Sunkopê

On the contrary, the notion of *sunkopê* is much better delimited and fitted for Galen's system. Moreover, he seems to have come up with a solution to the above-mentioned ongoing debate about the *locus affectus* of *sunkopê* being either in the stomach (as Celsus and the *Anonymus Parisinus* suggested) or in the heart (as Aretaeus posited). He distinguished two different kinds of *sunkopai*:

ἴδιον δὲ πάθος ἐν καρδίᾳ γίνεται κατὰ μὲν ἁπλῆν δυσκρασίαν πολλάκις ... ἕπονται δὲ πάλιν ταῖς τοιαύταις διαθέσεσιν αἱ καρδιακαὶ συγκοπαὶ, καθάπερ αἱ στομαχικαὶ ταῖς κατὰ τὸ τῆς κοιλίας στόμα ... αἱ διαθέσεις δ᾽ ἀμφοτέρων τῶν μορίων, τοῦ τε στόματος τῆς κοιλίας καὶ τῆς καρδίας, ἤτοι διὰ δυσκρασίαν μόνην ἰσχυρὰν ... εἰώθασι γίγνεσθαι ... ταῖς μεγάλαις δὲ [δυσκρασίαις]. *Loc. Aff. 5.2. K.VIII*: 302, 6–7; 10–17; 303, 3.

An intrinsic affection of the heart often occurs in simple [not compound] *duskrasia* [as well as in other diseases] ... Cardiac *sunkopê* follows these kind of conditions [*duskrasias* and the others], in the same way as stomachic *sunkopê* follows conditions affecting the mouth of the bowels ... The conditions of both parts, namely, the mouth of the bowels and the heart, ... tend to be produced ... either by a violent single *duskrasia* [or by the other diseases].

Despite this dual origin, namely, one affecting primarily the heart and the other one the mouth of the bowels,[5] Galen's theory of sympathies referred them both to their common corresponding *archê* in the heart. Thus, whether the condition originated in the stomach or in the heart, it needed to affect the latter (directly or sympathetically) in order to be considered as a *sunkopê*:

αἱ στομαχικαὶ δὲ συγκοπαὶ ... ἔκλυσιν ἐπιφέρουσιν, ἴσως δὲ καὶ τῆς δυσκρασίας αὐτοῦ διϊκνουμένης εἰς τὴν καρδίαν, ὡς κἀκείνης ἐν δυσκρασίᾳ γινομένης ἀθρόαν κατάπτωσιν ἀκολουθῆσαι τῆς δυνάμεως. *Loc. Aff. 5.6. K.VIII*: 342, 16–18; 343, 1–2.

Sunkopai of the stomach ... can bring about swoons. In like manner, when its imbalanced mixture [the *duskrasia* of the stomach] penetrates the heart to such an

---

[5] I interpret that *to stoma tês koilias* ('the mouth of the bowel') refers to the distal end of the oesophagus or proximal end of the stomach, which – as stated above – is still nowadays called 'cardia', hence the similarity with the heart and the possible confusion.

extent that it [the heart], too, becomes imbalanced [in *duskrasia*], a sudden collapse of capacities [that is, *sunkopê*] follows.

As regards the discussion on consciousness, the relevance of this issue stems from the fact that unlike the other forms of impaired consciousness (which were all related to some compromise of the *hêgemonikon* in the brain), in Galen's system *sunkopai* were never primarily a psychic condition regardless of its type. He even presents an experimental demonstration of this:

... ὅτι θλιβεισῶν μὲν ἢ τρωθεισῶν τῶν κατὰ τὸν ἐγκέφαλον κοιλῶν ὅλον τὸ ζῷον αὐτίκα γίνεται καρῶδες, οὐ μὴν ἀπόλλυται γε οὔτε ἡ κατὰ τὰς ἀρτηρίας οὔτε ἡ κατὰ τὴν καρδίαν κίνησις ... ἐγκεφάλου μὲν γὰρ πάσχοντος ἕτοιμον παραφρονῆσαί τε καὶ ἀκίνητον καὶ ἀναίσθητον γενέσθαι τὸ ζῷον, καρδίας δὲ συγκοπῆναι μὲν καὶ ἀπολέσθαι, τῶν προειρημένων δ᾽ οὐδὲ ἓν παθεῖν. *PHP. LCL III.5*: 210, 20–4; 30–3. *K.V*: 301–2.

... when the ventricles of the brain have been compressed or wounded, the whole animal becomes immediately drowsy (*karôdes*); however, neither does the movement in the arteries die nor [the movement] in the heart ... For if the brain is affected, the animal becomes readily delirious (*paraphronêsai*), paralysed (*akinêton*) and loses sensation (*anaisthêton*), whereas if the heart [is affected] it suffers *sunkopê* and dies, but [with] none of the aforementioned symptoms.

In this description – which suggests a strong anatomical basis – Galen very clearly opposes symptoms that he considered to be psychic (*karôdes, paraphronêsai, akinêton, anaisthêton*) to the non-psychic *sunkopê*. In line with his theory, the former occur in the brain and the latter in the heart.

Additionally, the contrast between *sunkopê* and swoons provides us with further details about how the former fitted into Galen's system.[6] In his *Method of healing*, *sunkopê* is defined as an ἡ συγκοπὴ κατάπτωσίς ... ἐστιν ὀξεῖα δυνάμεως ('acute collapse of the capacity'),[7] and some interesting tips are given to preserve such a capacity:

ἐξαίρετον δὲ εἰς ῥώμην δυνάμεως καὶ προφυλακὴν τοῦ μή ποτ᾽ ἐξαιφνίδιον ἐπιπεσεῖν παροξυσμὸν συγκοπτικὸν ἡ φυλακὴ τῆς εὐκρασίας ἐστί, πρῶτον μὲν τῶν τριῶν ἀρχῶν, ἔπειτα δὲ καὶ τῶν ἄλλων μορίων ὅσα τὰς ἀρχὰς εἰς συμπάθειαν

---

[6] This contrast suggests that Galen – like Aretaeus – also seems to have perceived *sunkopê* and swoons as similar or easily confusable phenomena needing differentiation.

[7] *MM LCL XII.5*: 264, 14–15. *K.X*: 837.

Galen's two ways of losing consciousness

ἐπισπᾶται ῥᾳδίως, οἷόν πέρ ἐστι καὶ τὸ τῆς γαστρὸς στόμα … συγκοπὰς ἐπιφέρον. ἡ μὲν οὖν προειρημένη διάθεσις τῶν ὠμῶν χυμῶν … ὀλέθριός τέ ἐστι καὶ συγκοπτική … καταπνίγεσθαι καὶ ἀλλοιοῦσθαι καὶ διαφθείρεσθαι τῆς κράσεως τὴν συμμετρίαν. οἱ μὲν γὰρ ὠμοὶ τρέφειν οὐ δύνανται πρὶν πεφθῆναι, οἱ δὲ πολλοὶ βαρύνουσιν· εἰ δ᾽ ἐμφράττουσι τὰς διαπνοὰς σβεννύουσι τὸ θερμόν· εἰ δὲ μήτ᾽ ἐμφράττοιεν μήτε βαρύνοιεν οὐ συγκοπὰς οὗτοί γε φέρουσιν, ἀλλὰ τὰς καλουμένας λειποψυχίας… *MM XII.5. LCL III:* 274, 5–22. *K.X:* 844–5.

It is crucial for the strength of the capacity and as a precaution to avoid ever falling into a sudden acute *sunkopê*, first to preserve the good balance (*eukrasia*) in the three principles (*archai*). Then, also, in the other parts that can easily attract them [the principles] towards *sympathy*, such as the mouth of the stomach … which can bring about *sunkopai*. Indeed, the aforementioned condition caused by uncooked humours … becomes deadly and predisposes one to *sunkopai* … by suffocating, altering and destroying the balance of the mixture. For those humours cannot nourish before they are concocted, but they do strain [the capacity] if they are abundant and quench the heat if they block the exhalations. If they neither block nor strain, such humours do not bring about syncopes, but the so-called fits of swooning (*leipopsuchia*)…

Again, a *duskrasia* in the stomach needed to affect the *archê* in the heart by *sympathy* in order to cause the condition. In this passage, moreover, the strong bodily components of *sunkopê* are highlighted in opposition to swoons. In a nutshell, the same kind of raw humours can produce either of them depending on their prevalent effect: if straining and blocking predominate, *sunkopê* occurs. Namely, *sunkopê* is caused by a cold *duskrasia* that manifests through clinically evident signs (quenched heat and blocked exhalations), whereas in *leipopsuchia* the humours only prevent nourishment, that is, they do not affect in a tangible way through their specific qualities. It is clear from the description that *sunkopê* fits perfectly well within Galen's system, where a distinct humoural action enables an adequate treatment to counterbalance the alteration, and a clear location determines the site of the treatment.

Naturally, once the *locus affectus* and the quality of the humours are found, therapy becomes straightforward:

ἐφ᾽ ὧν δὲ διὰ χολὴν ξανθὴν ἀδικήσασαν τὸ στόμα τῆς γαστρὸς ἡ συγκοπὴ γένοιτο, ψυχρὸν τούτοις χρὴ προσφέρειν τὸ ποτόν. οἶνον μέντοι τῇ φύσει θερμὸν εἰς ἀνάδοσιν ὁρμῶντα τοῖς συγκοπτομένοις ἅπασι δοτέον *MM XII.4. LCL III:* 252, 19–23. *K.X:* 830.

In cases where *sunkopê* is produced by yellow bile that harms the mouth of the stomach, it is necessary to administer a cold drink. For certain, wine should be given to all the patients who suffer *sunkopê*: due to its hot nature it stimulates the assimilation [of nourishment].

Again, the allopathic idea that opposites cure opposites is in play in the case of yellow bile: because it is hot it needs to be reversed by a cold drink. The use of wine is slightly different. I have mentioned above that *sunkopai* (as well as swoons) can be caused by uncooked humours, which do not nourish unless they are concocted. In this case wine is prescribed because – despite its hot nature – it helps to assimilate the nourishment. Further down Galen adds that ὁ μὲν μᾶλλον, ὁ δ᾽ ἧττον, ἅπαντες δ᾽ οὖν ... τονοῦσι ... τὸν στόμαχον ('all of them [the wines] ... strengthen the stomach to a greater or lesser degree').[8] Despite its apparently counteractive effect on the mixture, wine is indicated due to its favourable effect on the *locus affectus*.

From the analysis of Galen's approach to total loss of consciousness it emerges that – as opposed to the vagueness surrounding fainting – he conceived *sunkopê* as a condition anatomically unrelated to the other psychic diseases, due to its utter independence from the *hêgemonikon*. Unsurprisingly, and much like other authors, he seems to have associated it with a bodily condition, for in his view the heart was the seat of the spirited part of the *psuchê* in control over bodily functions (unlike the *hêgemonikon*, which governed cognition, rationality and thought).

Galen's tripartite soul and total loss of consciousness

The idea of the soul was a key concern for Galen in several works, and he devoted to it abundant philosophical reflection.[9] Very schematically, as we have seen, he organised the *psuchê* according

---

[8] *MM XII.4. LCL III*: 256, 6–8. *K.X*: 832.
[9] An in-depth description of Galenic psychology is beyond the scope of this analysis, and there is abundant scholarship that has addressed different aspects of it, particularly his physiological views regarding mental processes: Holmes (2013: 147–76) and Siegel (1973: 114–72); philosophical debates underlying his notion of the soul: Hankinson (1991: 194–217), Tracy (1976: 43–72), Tieleman (2003: 131–70) and von Staden (2002: 79–116). I will only explore here the way in which the *psuchê* is believed to interact and the extent to which it is involved in descriptions of total loss of consciousness.

to the Platonic model – into a rational, a spirited and a desiderative part – and described with thorough detail the subdivisions of the rational soul.[10] I have mentioned, so far, that this rational soul – and particularly its *hêgemonikon* – was variously compromised in both wakeful impaired consciousness and pathological sleep.

On the contrary, I have argued that from the two forms of total loss of consciousness – that is, *leipothumiê* and *sunkopê* – only the former was vaguely related to the ruling part of the soul. A possible element for such a link is the *pneuma*. Quite in line with Aretaeus, Galen's understanding of swoons involved the release of heat (*emphutos thermasia*),[11] the lack of nourishment[12] and also the loss of *pneuma*:

διὸ καὶ κενωθέν, ἄχρις ἂν αὖθις ἀθροισθῇ, τὴν μὲν ζωὴν οὐκ ἀφαιρεῖσθαι τὸ ζῷον, ἀναίσθητον δὲ καὶ ἀκίνητον ἐργάζεσθαι. καίτοι γε, εἴπερ ἦν αὐτὸ ἡ τῆς ψυχῆς οὐσία, συνδιεφθείρετ᾽ ἂν αὐτῷ κενουμένῳ παραχρῆμα τὸ ζῷον. *PHP. LCL VII.3:* 444, 8–11; 446, 13–15. *K.V:* 603; 606.

Therefore, when [the *pneuma*] is depleted, and until it is collected again, the life is not taken away from the animal, but lack of perceptions and movements result. For if [the *pneuma*] was indeed the substance of the soul, the animal would die immediately with its depletion.

Remarkably, in his view it is the *pneuma*, the primary element of the *psuchê* in the brain, but not the soul itself that dissipates in these conditions.[13] Of note is also the fact that he does not talk about *leipothumiê* but about total loss of perception and movement, which is virtually the same. This statement is quite strong when compared to all the other authors, who considered – in one way or another – that the entire soul was expelled during swoons. Additionally, two other interesting implications can be drawn from this passage: first and foremost, that this temporary loss of *pneuma* is compromising capacities in the rational soul, thereby linking total loss of consciousness to the other prototypical presentations; secondly, that although the soul referred to in this passage does not completely separate, it is still conceived as a life principle, for its loss is equated with death.

---

[10] *Symp. Diff. CMG (G).3:* 216, 19–20; 218, 1–6, 7–9. *K.VII:* 55–6.
[11] *Caus. Symp. II.5. K.VII:* 194, 9.   [12] *MM XII.5. LCL III:* 274, 19–20. *K.X:* 845.
[13] I have quoted above another passage where the loss of *pneuma* leaves the body in a state that is undistinguishable from a corpse (*PHP. LCL VII.3:* 446, 13–15. *K.V:* 606).

In other words, despite the contradictions that emerge from the various components altered during fainting, particularly the uncertainties regarding which specific part of the soul – or which *archê* – was affected (according to Galen the *pneuma* was associated with the rational *psuchê* in the brain, the blood to the spirited one located in the heart, and nourishment was related to the desiderative soul located in the liver), he was quite clear about the lethal effect of the loss of the *psuchê*.

On the other hand, *sunkopai* – whether they originated in the stomach or in the heart – ultimately compromised the *archê* in the heart (directly or by *sympathy*). In this regard, an interesting and rather puzzling comment appears in *On the causes of symptoms*. In the midst of a discussion on sweating Galen states:

μεταβαίνειν οὖν ἤδη καιρὸς ἐπὶ τοὺς ἱδρῶτας, ὑπὲρ ὧν εἴρηται μέν που τό γε τοσοῦτον ὡς ἀναλυομένης ἐνίοτε γίγνονται τῆς ἕξεως, καὶ καλεῖται τὸ πάθημα συγκοπή· τούτῳ δὲ ἐναντία κατάστασίς ἐστιν ἡ ἐν τοῖς κρισίμοις ἱδρῶσιν, ἐρρωμένην ἐνδεικνυμένοις, οὐ διαλυομένην τὴν φύσιν. *Symp. Caus. III.9. K.VII:* 252, 8–13.

It is time to address sweats, amongst which I have already discussed those that are produced to such a degree that they release the cohesion of the body (*hexis*). Such an affection is called *sunkopê*. The opposite condition to this is sweating in critical periods, which are demonstrative of good health, for nature (*phusis*) is not dissolved by them.

As we have seen with the post-Hellenistic sources, the association between sweating and *sunkopai* is very well documented. However, the terminology in this passage is particularly surprising for Galen. He is employing two Stoic concepts, *hexis* and *phusis*, which he does not normally use in relation to this condition. Furthermore, he seems to be considering them as synonyms, although according to Stoic philosophy they belong on different levels within the *scala naturae*.[14] Of note is the fact that both terms describe a low level of cohesion (characteristic of objects and plants), that is, always below *psuchê* (which allows perception and movement).[15] Therefore, despite the

---

[14] Annas (1992: 38).
[15] I also mentioned a similar confusion in Aretaeus, who used *phusis* and *psuchê* interchangeably. Nevertheless, this imperfection is less surprising in the context of Aretaeus' lax eclecticism, as opposed to Galen's precision in the use of terminology and his claim to expertise in philosophical matters.

uncharacteristic lack of philosophical accuracy, this might also be a hint of Galen's understanding of *sunkopê* as an affection alien to the rational *psuchê* and the psychic diseases. Similarly, in another passage, where he discusses stomachic *sunkopai*, he attributes it to *zôtikos tonos* ('weakness in the vital tension').[16] If this notion is in any way related to the Stoic *zôtikon pneuma*, then again we have an affection that compromises the key element of the spirited part of the soul located in the heart: namely, different from the *psuchikon pneuma* produced in the brain,[17] and hence different from the psychical conditions.

In summary, all the discussion above seems to suggest that the rational soul could be thought of as the linking element between the three presentations of impaired consciousness. However, it is less explicitly emphasised than in the other authors. Although there are hints that the loss of the main substance of the rational *psuchê* – *pneuma* – causes swoons, there are also allusions to the other parts of the soul, thereby connecting *leipothumiê* with *sunkopê*.

---

[16] *Loc. Aff. 5.1. K.VIII*: 301, 17.

[17] τοῦ μὲν δὴ ψυχικοῦ πνεύματος ἐναργῶς ἐδείξαμεν οἷον πηγήν τινα οὖσαν τὸν ἐγκέφαλον ... τοῦ δὲ ζωτικοῦ πνεύματος οὐχ ὁμοίως μὲν ἐναργῶς ἡ ἀπόδειξις ἦν, οὐ μὴν ἀπίθανόν γε κατά τε τὴν καρδίαν αὐτὸ καὶ τὰς ἀρτηρίας δοκεῖν περιέχεσθαι ('We have clearly demonstrated that the brain is like a certain fountain of psychic (*psuchikon*) pneuma ... The demonstration of vital (*zôtikon*) pneuma was not equally clear; however, it does not seem unlikely that it is contained in the heart and the arteries', *MM XII.5. LCL III*: 266, 20–6. *K.X*: 839).

CHAPTER 16

CONCLUDING REFLECTIONS ON THE IMPLICATION OF THE SOUL IN TOTAL LOSS OF CONSCIOUSNESS

Tieleman has accurately remarked that Aristotle had set the agenda of topics regarding psychology questions to be addressed and that several philosophers followed his lead.[1] We have seen throughout our discussion that a few doctors also addressed similar queries.

Schematically, the main issues under scrutiny – according to Tieleman's reading of Aristotle – were the existence of the soul as something in itself, its substance (*ousia*), the number and the type of its powers and its localisation in the body. As we have been seeing, all the medical writers under scrutiny (including the pre-Aristotelian ones) took the existence of the soul for granted. All of them started from the assumption that there is a soul and that it is a major player in impaired consciousness. The case of Galen should, perhaps, be nuanced because even if he insisted on how obvious it was, he did provide proof of the soul's existence in *On the doctrines of Hippocrates and Plato*. The substance was not a key issue, although some medical writers did attempt physiological explanations based on assumptions concerning the substance of the soul.[2] The most important concern for all these authors was the type of powers, the organisation of those powers and their localisation in the body. In other words, most doctors did take a position on each of the philosophical debates concerning the *psuchê*, but they only addressed the issues that were relevant to their practice. Unlike philosophers, they did not feel the need to justify all their assumptions. Galen, again, is the exception in this regard because he took part in medical and philosophical discussions alike.

---

[1] Tieleman (2003: 137).
[2] The Hippocratic treatise *On regimen* (35) emphasised the importance of fire and water to *phronêsis*; the *pneuma* pervades several Aretaean and Galenic explanations (although Galen is explicitly agnostic about the substance of the soul).

As far as total loss of consciousness is concerned, we have seen a unanimous understanding of this presentation as a near-death experience, which points towards an assimilation of the soul to a life force, as though during fainting the body was momentarily depleted of whatever kept it alive. Accordingly, we have seen that this 'life force', contained in the breath in the archaic literature (identified as *psuchê* and *thumos*), is represented among the Hippocratic doctors as a medicalised *psuchê* that temporarily abandons the body during swoons and permanently in death. Similarly, in Celsus' *On medicine*, it is the irrational part – the *anima* – of his dichotomous soul that reversibly separates during fainting and permanently departs with death. In Aretaeus this vital power, which the body becomes deprived of during total loss of consciousness, is construed as a tangle of ideas such as the heat of life of the body, the tension, the *pneuma* (all of them vaguely linked to his ill-defined *psuchê*). Finally, in Galen we should add the nuance that although total loss of consciousness was not strictly at the boundary between life and death (for in his account the soul did not actually separate during swoons – only the *pneuma* did), he did consider that the separation of the *psuchê* from the body was synonymous with dying, thereby equating his tripartite Platonic soul to a lifegiving entity.

Regarding the role of the *psuchê* as an abstract notion that provides a unifying theoretical common ground to the different presentations of impaired consciousness, it could be argued that this is certainly the case for the Hippocratic doctors. Amongst them, the all-encompassing *psuchê* – affected during total loss of consciousness – subsumed other constructs such as *sunesis, phronêsis, nous*, compromised in wakeful and drowsy impaired consciousness. Also in Celsus, the twin concepts *animus–anima* explain the different presentations of the condition. Thus, the rational component, *mens/animus/consilium*, is altered in delirium, whereas as suggested above, the degree of separation of the irrational *anima* – subordinated to the former – determines whether the patient faints (complete separation) or simply sleeps (partial separation). The case of Aretaeus is slightly different, because although there are common pathophysiological phenomena often associated with the different forms of impaired consciousness, he did not elaborate a consistent notion of the soul in his extant work, and his scattered allusions to it are often contradictory. There is, however, a unifying abstract concept that appears to be compromised in all the presentations of impaired consciousness. In line with Aretaeus' engagement with the debate around perceptions, it could be argued that *aisthêsis* plays in his argument a role similar to that of the soul in the other authors. This construct appears to be ubiquitously present and compromised in all these conditions: in swoons and sleep, perceptions are interrupted (more so in the former than in the latter, where pain can still be felt). In delirium, on the other hand, individuals perceive abnormal things while their thinking is intact (unlike other cognitive conditions – mental illness according to our current understanding – where the *gnômê* is compromised but perceptions are intact). In Galen, finally, the soul is again a common component of the different presentations of impaired consciousness: its rational part in delirium and sleep, and all three components – especially the spirited soul – in the different forms of fainting.

In terms of interaction between body and soul (and the instrumentalist versus materialist debate), our authors' understanding of impaired consciousness suggests that all these medical models of the soul had a strong functional component. From the Hippocratic texts onwards we can see that their grasp of diseases where consciousness was impaired is based on the compromise of certain capacities (or the abolition of all of them in cases of fainting), and that medical debates focused on which those capacities were, how they were grouped (or subsumed into larger constructs) and where exactly in the body they were located.

From a chronological point of view one can see a progressive identification and isolation of such functions, particularly after the anatomical Hellenistic developments, where perceptions and movement started to play a more central role in most explanations, thereby reducing the relevance of more vague Hippocratic concepts, such as *sunesis, phronêsis, nous*. Simultaneously, the idea of a ruling part also reduced the debates on locations to the cardiocentric versus the encephalocentric stance. Notwithstanding all these simplifications, the tension between body and soul remained unchanged, in the sense that conditions like delirium, sleep and *leipothumiê* tended to be regarded as diseases where the soul (or its rational part) was primarily affected and, through it, the body (in other words, an instrumentalist stance), whereas *sunkopê* was mainly conceived as a bodily condition that interrupted several capacities that belonged to or depended on the integrity of the soul (the materialistic view). Of course, it is our current understanding of consciousness as a continuum and of syncopes as a form of swoon that allows us to understand this distinction as artificial.

CONCLUSIONS

In the Introduction I set out to explore accounts of impaired consciousness in ancient medical texts along two axes. In the longitudinal thematic one, I aimed to contrast the different approaches to the topic against their respective medical contexts and to establish relationships between texts, authors and periods. The transversal axis, on the other hand, focused on how the development of ideas and debates around impaired consciousness illuminates our understanding of other concepts about ancient medicine in general and about the authors referred to in particular. In summarising the main findings of this research I will first focus on the transversal axis, and then I shall add my final remarks about impaired consciousness itself.

Transversal axis: what has the analysis of consciousness revealed about the sources?

The Hippocratic beginnings: a limited terminology for a multiplicity of symptoms

The Hippocratic doctors were a self-recognised group that shared – despite their heterogeneity – a set of ideas[1] for which they developed a particular technical language that enabled them to claim authority and differentiate themselves from rivals and competitors. However, the degree of development and level of technicality of their vocabulary remains contested.[2] In this context, my hypothesis about these writers' use of partial synonymy in discussing forms of impaired consciousness provided a feasible solution to some ongoing terminological disputes, even if it has challenged most of the recent scholarship around

---

[1] Cross (2018).   [2] Dean-Jones (2003).

this particular semantic field. Contrary to the predominant view,[3] this analysis suggests that both in terms of usage and meaning, most of the words utilised by the Hippocratic authors to talk about delirium are often interchangeable (much like our own contemporary medical vocabulary, and despite their apparent variety and multiplicity). Furthermore, this partial synonymy is paralleled by a similar (though not identical) phenomenon that involves the terminology for HOFs. Indeed, the concepts that these medical writers used to refer to the mental and cognitive capacities compromised during impaired consciousness are also more or less equivalent throughout the texts.

The relevance of these findings is that they point towards a rudimentary notion that pervades various conditions within the whole spectrum of consciousness (as we nowadays construe it), and that is shared by a large number of Hippocratic authors. This, ultimately, suggests that these writers understood that certain related conditions (which we can liken to our understanding of impaired consciousness) occur when certain capacities (which are subsumed in our idea of consciousness) are disturbed. As exemplified, descriptions of all three clinical presentations, as well as the recovery terminology, are permeated by this embryonic idea akin to our notion of consciousness. Stated in a complementary manner: delirium, sleep, swoons and their termination – in other words, coming round and waking up – are discussed by the Hippocratic doctors using a similar group of words, compounds of such words and phrasal terms in which those words are the noun head. Such a coincidence suggests that all the conditions under scrutiny belonged in the same semantic field, and therefore were related in these authors' conception. Hence, it is legitimate to posit that one of the notions that provides a certain unity to the plurality of the Hippocratic discourses is a shared underlying seminal idea of consciousness, which they considered to be compromised during the affections that we identified as prototypical of impaired consciousness.

---

[3] Particularly Thumiger (2013), but also di Benedetto (1986) and Pigeaud (1987).

Post-Hellenistic sources: organisation of knowledge and focus on nosology

The analysis expanded on the well-described multi-layered nature of the post-Hellenistic treatises[4] by revealing the way in which the authors under scrutiny dealt with the numerous voices available to them. It emerged that despite the evident differences between encyclopaedic and eclectic approaches, both have shown significant inconsistencies in terms of explaining the mechanisms underlying diseases. Indeed, Aretaeus and Celsus alike (and also the authors of the *Introduction*, the *Medical definitions* and the *Anonymus Parisinus*) privileged comprehensive dichotomous taxonomic systems – sometimes even overlooking clinical descriptions – over consistency in their understanding of the pathophysiological mechanisms involved. These findings are in line with the proliferation of diseases, concepts and the primacy of taxonomical distinctions in this period.[5]

Accordingly, starting from the diversity of post-Hellenistic medicine in terms of practitioners, theories, classifications and definitions,[6] the analysis points towards a fragmentation of impaired consciousness into smaller unities, that is, more specific diseases (as compared to the broader and vaguer Hippocratic syndromes). This phenomenon was favoured by the introduction of new nosological entities, by a more thorough delimitation of existing ones and by the development of specific treatments for each of them. Forcing the mutable reality of impaired consciousness into a strict theoretical framework inevitably distanced the medical writers from empiric clinical observation and diminished the perceived connection among the three prototypical clinical presentations. Nevertheless, the evidence suggests that despite these theoretical constraints the authors were able to relate delirium to sleep and swoons, which points towards an underlying shared idea of impaired consciousness.

---

[4] Longrigg (1993: 182), Nutton (2013a: 142).
[5] Perhaps Aretaeus' case should be nuanced in this regard, for he often included an ad hoc explanation when his clinical findings failed to adhere to the nosological classifications.
[6] Nutton (1995: 44–5).

Conclusions

Celsus and corpuscular theories

The inquiry into impaired consciousness suggests the significant influence of corpuscular theoretical systems in *On medicine*, which – to my knowledge – had never been mentioned before, despite the multiple scholarly studies on the influences and sources that its author used.[7] In analogy to what Beagon has remarked concerning Pliny's Stoicism, it is possible to envisage an Epicurean/Asclepiadean background influence in Celsus, which pervades his understanding of several processes. It is never explicit, and it probably reflects a common phenomenon among the intellectual Roman elites, namely, the adoption of a 'philosophical veneer' or an 'intellectual wallpaper' that conditioned their world view.[8] The parallels found between Lucretius' *On nature* and Celsus' *On medicine* suggest the above.

Two important implications can be drawn from this finding. On the one hand, it offers further support to Polito's and Leith's ideas about the Epicurean influences on Asclepiades[9] (thereby opposing Vallance's hypothesis).[10] On the other, it should warn us – as readers of the treatise – that although Celsus claims to look for the 'middle way' and explicitly tries to be inclusive of different positions, we must be careful in our reading of his text, because there is a bias towards a materialistic corpuscular understanding of certain processes. In other words, his *media quodammodo diversas inter sententias* leans towards this Epicurean/Asclepiadean view of the workings of the human body in conditions where consciousness is impaired. It might be worth exploring – in future endeavours – whether this stance is also present in relation to other affections, where the interaction between body, mind and soul is not at stake.

Aretaeus and lax eclecticism

In the case of Aretaeus, most scholarly controversies have focused on his sectarian affiliation. I reject the predominant hypothesis to group him among the Pneumatists[11] or to simply highlight his

[7] Scarborough (1993), von Staden (1994a), Stok (1993), Mudry (1993).
[8] Beagon (2005: 16).   [9] Polito (2006), Leith (2009).   [10] Vallance (1990).
[11] Verbeke (1945), Stannard (1964), Oberhelman (1993).

200

coincidences with the Hippocratic authors,[12] and propose instead to overcome the debate by focusing on his method. By looking at the way in which he explained the different processes and occurrences in diseases with impaired consciousness, it would appear that he drew from an abundance of theories available to explain these phenomena without strictly sticking to any of them. Thus, 'lax eclecticism' emerges as an alternative solution to a dispute that cannot be settled with the evidence that we currently have about the Pneumatic and Eclectic sects. The notion of lax eclecticism, therefore, deflects the focus of the sectarian debate onto a methodological one and reflects Aretaus' imperfect attempt at compiling a coherent, consistent and comprehensive explanation for diseases and their mechanisms, by taking components from different – and often contradictory – sources.[13] It would seem that through this eclectic approach he addressed competing sectarian voices and made his own choices, thereby establishing his authority.

Moreover, because lax eclecticism presupposes the inclusion of elements from such different theoretical frameworks, it reveals – on the one hand – that impaired consciousness was being actively debated; that is, it was a focus of interest for physicians, and no single answer had been unanimously considered as satisfactory. On the other hand, the multiplicity of theories addressed illustrates the extent to which the medical discourse incorporated ideas debated in other disciplines – particularly philosophy – in order to understand and elucidate its clinical findings. Indeed, most of Aretaeus' explanations about impaired consciousness are strongly influenced by contemporary philosophical debates on the relation between sensory perceptions and the reality behind them, as Pigeaud has illustrated.[14]

Galen: a totalising approach

The present analysis sheds light on some specific details about the workings of the body and the mind in Galen's comprehensive medical

---

[12] Pigeaud (2004), McDonald (2009b), Murphy (2013).
[13] I consider it imperfect because it was neither coherent nor consistent.
[14] Pigeaud (1987: 95–9).

Conclusions

system. At the same time, it illustrates the level of coherence, consistency and explanatory power that it achieved. As several scholars have pointed out, he was able to frame the conditions within a carefully articulated system that combined well-established theories (humours, qualities, elements) with cutting-edge advances in medical knowledge (particularly anatomical).[15] Contrary to Pigeaud's view,[16] I have suggested that he also succeeded in rationally connecting – without strong contradictions – the pathophysiological mechanisms with the therapy for such conditions. In this way, even when he proposed the same treatment as his competitors,[17] he was able to claim authority by explaining the rationality of his choice (an ability which his opponents lacked).

In terms of Galen's take on mental affections, the notion of impaired consciousness offers a more comprehensive model for the conditions that Devinant 'tacitly identified as a nosologic space', where the soul – more specifically its *hegêmonikon* – was affected.[18] I partially agree with his idea that (what I claim to be) delirium is sometimes grouped together with psychiatric conditions – as I described in relation to *mania* (but not with *melancholia*). However, the present study has illustrated how other conditions – such as abnormal sleep and fainting, which we nowadays associate with impaired consciousness – were equally related to a compromise in the rational soul.

On the other hand, the analysis also uncovered some limits to the system that are not usually discussed by the scholarship. Because Galen was mainly focused on organs and quantities as well as the qualities of the mixtures, he was less detailed in his reflections on specific conditions. Hence, his model was weaker than the post-Hellenistic ones in distinguishing impaired consciousness from some neurological and psychiatric diseases (the case of the paralysed child among diseases of the *hêgemonikon* and the lack of attention to *mania* illustrate this shortcoming). Similarly, the strict boundaries that his view presupposed sometimes obscured certain continuities. Such is the case of the total separation that he articulates between normal and abnormal sleep.

[15] Schöner (1964), Nutton (1995: 66–9), Mattern (2013).   [16] Pigeaud (2008: 582).
[17] Frede (1987: 262).   [18] Devinant (2020: 299).

Longitudinal thematic axis: advantages of exploring impaired consciousness

Impaired consciousness – a notion scarcely referred to in recent scholarship – emerges from this analysis as a powerful concept that provides valid answers to several controversial debates and groups together three clinical presentations (delirium, sleep and fainting) that had not been perceived so far by researchers as connected entities. As a result, the ideas about the role of the mind and the soul – and their relation to the body – which emerge from their analysis as a whole had been so far disregarded. Up until now, such debates had been mainly addressed by focusing only on delirium and mental illness.[19]

Moreover, the notion of impaired consciousness condenses in itself a tension between two conceptual movements in opposite directions, which mirrors a dichotomy present in medical thought more generally. On the one hand, there is an attempt to explain the diseases through increasingly concrete and limited elements that the medical systems can easily address, such as humours, secretions, qualities, obstructions. On the other, there is a tendency to create progressively abstract notions (the *gnômê*, the *psuchê*, the *hêgemonikon*, etc.), which subsume the whole phenomenon in complex theoretical systems. The doctors navigate these tensions, but it is always the successful treatment to regulate the concrete altered bodily component that prevails over the perfectly functioning abstract model.

In this sense, this medically informed approach to psychology-related debates has highlighted some aspects that are absent from purely philosophical treatises. Regardless of the specific model that each author envisaged, any speculation is ultimately subordinated to the pragmatic approach of medicine. Doctors only considered their theories to be valid if they were useful in guiding therapy, and the better the treatment the stronger the theory. No matter how philosophically minded the author might have been, the theory could only be validated by the clinical outcomes; that is, logic always yielded to the results. In other words, although

---

[19] A few examples are Pigeaud (1981), di Benedetto (1986), Singer (1992), Gundert (2000), von Staden (2002), van der Eijk (2005), King (2006), Devinant (2020).

theoretical coherence was valued, some philosophical contradiction could be tolerated (even by Galen as his use of *hexis* and
phusis suggests) as long as there were positive outcomes.

Finally, with a view to organising these ideas in relation to
current scholarly constructs, we should perhaps regard impaired
consciousness as a distinct category that is independent from
mental illness even if it shares fuzzy edges with it. Naturally,
within each of these categories a number of nosological entities
along with non-nosological processes (such as healthy sleep) can
be singled out, which are also sometimes difficult to separate from
one another, because they too share some fuzzy edges. Apart from
avoiding misleadingly applying modern concepts to ancient constructs, the advantage of this framework is that it better reflects the
fluidity of the boundaries not only between the concrete diseases
concerned, but also between the notions of health and disease,
wakefulness and sleep and even between life and death in the
world of ancient medical discourse.

BIBLIOGRAPHY

Primary sources

Anonymus Parisinus

Anon. Paris. *Anonymi medici de morbis acutis et chroniis. Anonymus Parisinus.* Edit. with commentary by I. Garofalo; translated into English by B. Fuchs. Leiden: Brill. 1997.

Aretaeus of Cappadocia

On the causes, symptoms and cure of acute and chronic diseases. CMG 2. Edit. K. Hude. Leipzig: Teubner. 1923.

SA I *De causis et signis acutorum morborum I (H.I).*
SA II *De causis et signis acutorum morborum II (H.II).*
SD I *De causis et signis diuturnorum morborum I (H.III).*
SD II *De causis et signis diuturnorum morborum II (H.IV).*
CA I *De curatione acutorum morborum I (H.V).*
CA II *De curatione acutorum morborum II (H.VI).*
CD I *De curatione diuturnorum morborum I (H.VII).*
CD II *De curatione diuturnorum morborum II (H.VIII).*

Aristophanes

Nu. *Nubes. Aristophanes, Clouds.* Edit. by F.W. Hall, W.M. Geldart. Oxford: Oxford University Press. 1907.

Aristotle

DA *De anima. Aristotle, On the soul.* Introduction, translation and notes by R. Polansky. New York: Cambridge University Press. 2007.
EN *Ethica Nicomachea. Aristotle, Nicomachean ethics.* English translation by H. Rackham. (Loeb Classical Library). London: Heinemann. 1934.

Bibliography

GA *De generatione animalium. Aristotle, Generation of animals.* Translated by A.L. Peck (Loeb Classical Library). Cambridge, MA: Harvard University Press. 1942.

GC *De generatione et corruptione. Aristotle, On coming-to-be and passing-away.* Translated by E.S. Forster and D.J. Furley. (Loeb Classical Library). London: Heinemann. 1955.

PA *De partibus animalium. Aristotle, Parts of animals.* Translated by A.L. Peck and E.S. Forster. (Loeb Classical Library). Cambridge, MA: Harvard University Press. 1961.

Insomn. *De insomniis. Aristotle, On dreams* in *Petits traités d'histoire naturelle.* Edited and translated by R. Mugnier. Paris: Les belles lettres. 1953.

Somn. et Vig. *De somno et vigilia. Aristotle, On sleep and waking* in *Petits traités d'histoire naturelle.* Edited and translated by R. Mugnier. Paris: Les belles lettres. 1953.

Caelius Aurelianus

Aur. Acut. *Acutae passiones. Caelius Aurelianus, On acute diseases and chronic diseases.* Edited and translated by I.E. Drabkin. Chicago: University of Chicago Press. 1950.

Celsus

Med. *De medicina. C. Aulus Celsus, On medicine.* Edit. by W.G. Spencer. (Loeb Classical Library). Cambridge, MA and London: Harvard University Press; Heinemann. 1960.

Cicero

Div. *De divinatione. Cicero, On divination.* Translated by W.A. Falconer. (Loeb Classical Library). Cambridge, MA; London: Harvard University Press. 1923.

TD *Tusculanae disputationes. Cicero, Tusculan disputations.* Translated by J.E. King. (Loeb Classical Library, Rev. ed.) Cambridge, MA: Harvard University Press. 1945.

Corpus Hippocraticum: texts from the Hippocratic corpus

Acut. *De victu acutorum. On regimen in acute diseases. Hippocrate CUF 4.2: Du régime des maladies aiguës.* Edit. by A. Joly. Paris: Les belles lettres. 1972.

Bibliography

Acut. Sp. *De victu acutorum, Sp. On regimen in acute diseases*, in *Hippocrates* (Loeb Classical Library. Vol. 6). Edit. by P.B. Potter. London and Cambridge, MA: Heinemann. 1988.

Aer. *De aere, aquis, locis. On airs, waters and places. Hippocrate CUF 2.2: Airs, eaux, lieux.* Edit. J. Jouanna. Paris: Les belles lettres. 1996.

Aff. *De affectionibus. On affections*, in *Hippocrates* (Loeb Classical Library. Vol. 5). Edit. P. Potter. London and Cambridge, MA: Heinemann. 1988.

Aph. *Aphorisimi. Aphorisms,* in *Hippocrates* (Loeb Classical Library. Vol. 4). Edit. W.H.S. Jones. London and Cambridge, MA: Heinemann. 1967.

Art. *De arte. Hippocrates, On the art of medicine.* Edit. J.E. Mann. Leiden: Brill. 2012.

Artic. *De articulis. On joints*, in *Hippocrates* (Loeb Classical Library. Vol. 3). Edit. E.T. Withington. London and Cambridge, MA: Heinemann. 1928.

C. *De glandulis. On glands. The Hippocratic treatise On glands.* Edit. E. M. Craik, edition, translation, introduction and notes. Leiden: Brill. 2009.

Coac. *Coacae praenotiones. Coan prenotions*, in *Hippocrates* (Loeb Classical Library. Vol. 9). Edit. P. Potter. London and Cambridge, MA: Heinemann. 2010.

Epid. I. *Epidemiarum I. Epidemics book 1. Hippocrate CUF 4.1: Epidémies I et III.* Edit. J. Jouanna. Paris: Les belles lettres. 2016.

Epid. II. *Epidemiarum II. Epidemics book 2*, in *Hippocrates* (Loeb Classical Library. Vol. 7). Edit. W.D. Smith. London and Cambridge, MA: Heinemann. 1994.

Epid. III. *Epidemiarum III. Epidemics book 3. Hippocrate CUF 4.1: Epidémies I et III.* Edit. J. Jouanna. Paris: Les belles lettres. 2016.

Epid. IV. *Epidemiarum IV. Epidemics book 4*, in *Hippocrates* (Loeb Classical Library. Vol. 7). Edit. W.D. Smith. London and Cambridge, MA: Heinemann. 1994.

Epid. V. *Epidemiarum V. Epidemics book 5, Hippocrate CUF 4.3: Epidémies V et VII.* Edit. J. Jouanna. Paris: Les belles lettres. 2000.

Epid. VI. *Epidemiarum VI. Epidemics book 6*, in *Hippocrates* (Loeb Classical Library. Vol. 7). Edit. W.D. Smith. London and Cambridge, MA: Heinemann. 1994.

Epid. VII. *Epidemiarum VI. Epidemics book 7, Hippocrate CUF 4.3: Epidémies V et VII.* Edit. J. Jouanna. Paris: Les belles lettres. 2000.

Flat. *De flatibus. On breaths. Hippocrate CUF 5.1: Des vents – De l'art.* Edit. J. Jouanna. Paris: Les belles lettres. 1988.

Hum. *De humoribus. On humours. CMG 1.3, 1.* Edit. O. Overwien. Berlin: Akademie Verlag. 2014.

Int. *De internis affectionibus. On internal affections*, in *Hippocrates* (Loeb Classical Library. Vol. 6). Edit. P. Potter. London and Cambridge, MA: Heinemann. 1988.

Morb. I. *De morbis I. On diseases 1*, in *Hippocrates* (Loeb Classical Library. Vol. 5). Edit. P. Potter. London and Cambridge, MA: Heinemann. 1988.

Bibliography

Morb. II. *De morbis II. On diseases 2*, in *Hippocrates* (Loeb Classical Library. Vol. 5). Edit. P. Potter. London and Cambridge, MA: Heinemann. 1988.

Morb. III. *De morbis III. On diseases 3*, in Hippocrates (Loeb Classical Library. Vol. 6). Edit. P. Potter. London and Cambridge, MA: Heinemann. 1988.

Morb. IV. *De morbis IV. On diseases 4*, in *Hippocrates* (Loeb Classical Library. Vol. 10). Edit. P. Potter. London and Cambridge, MA: Heinemann. 2012.

Morb. Sacr. *De morbo sacro. On the sacred disease. Hippocrate CUF 2.3: La maladie sacrée*. Edit. J. Jouanna. Paris: Les belles lettres. 2003.

Mul. I. *De morbis mulierum I. On diseases of women 1*, in *Hippocrates* (Loeb Classical Library. Vol. 11). Edit. P. Potter. London and Cambridge, MA: Heinemann. 2018.

Mul. II. *De morbis mulierum II. On diseases of women 2*, in *Hippocrates* (Loeb Classical Library. Vol. 11). Edit. P. Potter. London and Cambridge, MA: Heinemann. 2018.

De Nat. Hom. *De natura hominis. On the nature of man. CMG I.1,3.* Edit. J. Jouanna. Berlin: Preussische Akademie der Wissenschaften. 2002.

Prog. *Prognosticum. Prognostic. Hippocrate CUF 3.1: Prognostic.* Edit. J. Jouanna. Paris: Les belles lettres. 2013.

Prorrh. I. *Prorrheticus I. Prorrhetic 1*, in *Hippocrates* (Loeb Classical Library. Vol. 8). Edit. P. Potter. London and Cambridge, MA: Heinemann. 1995.

VC *De vulneribus in capite. On head wounds. CMG 1,4,1.* Edit. M. Hanson. Berlin: Akademie Verlag. 1999.

Vict. *De victu. On regimen. CMG 1,2,4.* Edit. A. Joly and S. Byl. Berlin: Akademie Verlag. 1984.

Virg. *De virginum morbis. On diseases of girls. Hippocrate CUF XII.4: Maladies des jeunes filles.* Edit. F. Bourbon. Paris: Les belles lettres. 2017.

VM *De vetere medicina. On ancient medicine.* Edit. M.J. Schiefsky with translation, introduction and commentary. Leiden: Brill. 2005.

Epicurus

Ep. Hdt. *Epicurus' letter to Herodotus.* Edit. A.A Long and D.N. Sedley in *The Hellenistic philosophers*. Cambridge: Cambridge University Press. 1987.

Euripides

Eur. fr. *Euripides fragments. Euripides. fragments: Aegeus-Meleager* (Loeb Classical Library. Vol. 7). Edit. R. Kannicht. Translation by C. Collard and M. Cropp. London and Cambridge, MA: Heinemann. 2008.

Hipp. *Hippolytos. Euripides, Hippolytos.* Edit. by J. Diggle. Oxford: Oxford University Press. 1984.

Bibliography

Galen of Pergamum: texts from the Galenic corpus

Ars. Med. *Ars medica. The art of medicine. Galen CUF.II.* Edit. V. Boudon-Millot. Paris: Les belles lettres, 2000. (Kuhn I, 305–412.)

Caus. Morb. *De causis morborum. On the causes of diseases*, in *Claudii Galeni opera omnia*. Edit. C.G. Kuhn (1821). VII, 1–41. Cambridge: Cambridge University Press. 2011.

Caus. Puls. *De causis pulsuum. On the causes of the pulses*, in *Claudii Galeni opera omnia*. Edit. C.G. Kuhn (1821). IX, 1–204. Cambridge: Cambridge University Press. 2011.

Caus. Symp. *De symptomatum causis. On the causes of symptoms*, in *Claudii Galeni opera omnia*. Edit. C.G. Kuhn (1821). VII, 85–272. Cambridge: Cambridge University Press. 2011.

Cris. *De crisibus. On crises,* in *Claudii Galeni opera omnia*. Edit. C.G. Kuhn (1821). IX, 550–760. Cambridge: Cambridge University Press. 2011.

Hipp. Com. *De comate secundum Hippocratem. On the Coma according to Hippocrates. CMG V9,2.* Edit. I. Mewaldt, H. Diels and I. Heeg. Leipzig: Preussische Akademie der Wissenschaften. 1915. (Kuhn VII, 643–65.)

Hipp. Elem. *De elementis ex Hippocratis sententia. On the elements according to Hippocrates. CMG V1,2.* Edit. P. de Lacy. Berlin: Preussische Akademie der Wissenschaften. 1996. (Kuhn I, 413–508.)

Lib. Prop. *De libris propriis. On my own books. Galen. CUF.I.* Edit. V. Boudon-Millot. Paris: Les belles lettres. 2007. (Kuhn XIX, 8–48.)

Loc. Aff. *De locis affectis. On the affected parts: Books I and II*, in *CMG V6,1,1.* Edit. F. Gärtner. Berlin: Preussische Akademie der Wissenschaften (Kuhn VIII, 1–135.)

Books III to VI in *Claudii Galeni opera omnia*. Edit. C.G. Kuhn (1821). VIII, 136–452. Cambridge: Cambridge University Press. 2011.

MM *Methodos medendi. The method of medicine*. Edit. I. Johnston, G.H.R. Horsley. Cambridge, MA: Harvard University Press. 2011. (Kuhn X, 1–1021.)

Morb. Diff. *De morborum differentiis. On the distinction of diseases*, in *Claudii Galeni opera omnia*. Edit. C.G. Kuhn (1821). VI, 836–80. Cambridge: Cambridge University Press. 2011.

PHP *De placitis Hippocratis et Platonis. On the doctrines of Hippocrates and Plato. CMG V4,1,2.* Edit. P. De Lacy. Leipzig: Preussische Akademie der Wissenschaften. 1978. (Kuhn V, 181–805.)

QAM *Quod animi mores corporis temperamenta sequuntur. The capacities of the soul follow the mixtures of the body*, in *Claudii Galeni Pergami scripta minora*. Edit. I. Mueller. 2, 32–79. Leipzig: Teubner. 1891. (Kuhn IV, 767–822.)

Symp. Diff. *De symptomatum differentiis. On the distinction of symptoms. CMG V5,1.* Edit. B. Gundert. Berlin: Akademie Verlag. 2009. (Kuhn VII, 42–84.)

Bibliography

UP De usu partium. On the use of parts, in *Claudii Galeni opera omnia*. Edit. C. G. Kuhn (1821). III, 1–933. Cambridge: Cambridge University Press. 2011.

'Hippocrates': see Corpus Hippocraticum

Homer

Il. The Iliad. Homer. Translated by A.T. Murray, revised by W.F. Wyatt. (Loeb Classical Library.) London and Cambridge, MA: Harvard University Press. 1999.

Lucretius

Rer. nat. De rerum natura. Lucretius, On nature. Edit. M.F. Smith. Translated by W.H.D. Rouse. (Loeb Classical Library.) Cambridge, MA: Harvard University Press. 1975.

Plato

Tim. Timaeus. Plato. Timée, in *Oeuvres complètes* (Vol. 10). Edited and translated by A.R. Rivaud. Paris: Les belles lettres. 1925 (1970).

Pliny the elder

Nat. Hist. Naturalis historia. Pliny, Natural history. Translation by H. Rackham. (Loeb Classical Library.) London and Cambridge, MA: Harvard University Press. 1962.

Pseudo-Galen

Int. Introductio siue Medicus. Pseudo-Galien, Le médecin, introduction. Edit. C. Petit. Paris: Les belles lettres. 2009.
Def. Med. Definitiones medicae. Pseudo-Galen, Medical definitions, in *Claudii Galeni opera omnia*. Edit. C.G. Kuhn (1821). XIX, 346–462. Cambridge: Cambridge University Press. 2011.

Rufus of Ephesus

QM Rufus of Ephesus, Quaestiones medicales. Edit. H. Gärtner. Leipzig: Teubner. 1970.

Bibliography

Thucydides

Thuc. *Thucydides. Thucydides, History of the Peloponnesian war.* Translated by C.F. Smith (Loeb Classical Library). Cambridge, MA; London: Harvard University Press. 1928.

Valerius Maximus

Dicta et facta memorabilia. *Valerius Maximus, Memorable sayings and doings.* Edit. by D.R. Shackleton Bailey. (Loeb Classical Library.) London and Cambridge, MA: Harvard University Press. 2000.

Secondary sources

Aitchinson J. 1994, *Words in the mind: an introduction to the mental lexicon.* 2nd Ed. Oxford and Cambridge, MA: Blackwell.

Albrecht M. 1994, *Eklektik. Eine Begriffsgeschichte mit Hinweisen auf die Philosophie- und Wissenschaftsgeschichte.* Stuttgart-Bad Cannstatt: Frommann-Holzboog.

André J.M. 1987, *Être médecin à Rome.* Paris: Les belles lettres.

André J.M. 2006, *La médecine à Rome.* Paris: Tallandier.

Annas J. 1992, *Hellenistic philosophy of mind.* Berkeley: University of California Press.

Asmis E. 2016, 'Galen's *De indolentia* and the creation of a personal philosophy' in *Galen's De indolentia: essays on a newly discovered letter.* Edit. C.K. Rothschild and T.W. Thompson. Tübingen: Mohr Siebeck. 127–42.

Aubert V. and White H. 1959, 'Sleep: a sociological interpretation' in *Acta Sociologica* 4(2): 46–54.

Bailey C. 1947, *De rerum natura: libri sex. Titi Lucreti Cari.* Edit. C. Bailey, with prolegomena, critical apparatus, translation and commentary. Oxford: Clarendon.

Banu I. 1983, 'Les Hippocratiques de l'âge classique et l'anthropophilosophie' in *Formes de pensée dans la collection hippocratique: actes du IVe colloque international hippocratique* (Lausanne, 21–26 September 1981). Edit. F. Lasserre and P. Mudry. Geneva: Librairie Droz. 77–84.

Barker E.T.E. 2011, 'The Iliad's big swoon: a case of innovation within the epic tradition?' in *Trends in Classics* 3: 1–17.

Bartos H. 2015, *Philosophy and dietetics in the Hippocratic On regimen.* Leiden: Brill.

Beagon M. 2005, *The elder Pliny on the human animal: natural history book 7.* Oxford: Clarendon Press.

Bibliography

Benett S. 2013, "'Carving nature at the joints": the dream of a perfect classification of mental illness' in *Mental disorders in the classical world*. Edit. W.V. Harris. Leiden and Boston: Brill. 27–40.

Block N. 2002, 'Some concepts of mind' in *Philosophy of mind: classical and contemporary readings'*. Edit. D.J. Chalmers. Oxford: Oxford University Press. 206–19.

Boehm I. 2002, 'Inconscience et insensibilité dans la collection hippocratique' in *Le normal et le pathologique dans la Collection hippocratique: actes du Xe colloque hippocratique* (Nice, 6–9 October 1999). Nice-Sophia Antipolis: Publications de la Faculté des Lettres, Arts et Sciences humaines. 257–70.

Boudon-Millet V. 2000, *Galien: Exhortation à la médecine, Art médical* (Tome II). Paris: Les belles lettres.

Boudon-Millet V. 2013, 'What is a mental illness, and how can it be treated? Galen's reply as a doctor and philosopher' in *Mental disorders in the classical world*. Edit. W.V. Harris. Leiden: Brill. 129–46.

Bremmer J. 1983, *The early Greek concept of the soul*. Princeton, NJ: Princeton University Press.

Brunt L. and Steger B. 2003, 'Introduction: into the night and the world of sleep' in *Night-time and sleep in Asia and the West: exploring the dark side of life*. Edit. L. Brunt and B. Steger. Vienna: Abteilung für Japanologie des Instituts für Ostasienwissenschaften der Universität Wien. 1–24.

Burkeman O. 2014, 'Why can't the world's greatest minds solve the mystery of consciousness' in the *Guardian*: http://www.theguardian.com/science/2015/jan/21/-sp-why-cant-worlds-greatest-minds-solve-mystery-consciousness (last accessed 7 November 2019).

Byl S. 1998, 'Sommeil et insomnie dans le Corpus Hippocraticum' in *Revue Belge de Philosophie et d'Histoire*. 76(1): 31–6.

Byl S. 2002, 'Le vocabulaire de l'intelligence dans le chapitre 35 du livre I du traité du régime' in *Revue de Philologie, de Littérature et d'Histoire Anciennes*. 76: 217–24.

Carmel D. and Spreavak M. 2015, 'What is consciousness?' in *Philosophy and the sciences for everyone*. Edit. M. Massimi. London: Routledge. 103–22.

Chalmers D.J. 2010, *The character of consciousness*. Oxford: Oxford University Press.

Clark P.A. and Rose M.L. 2013, 'Psychiatric disability and the Galenic medical matrix' in *Disabilities in Roman antiquity: disparate bodies a capite ad calcem*. Edit. C. Laes, C. Goodey and M. Lynn Rose. Leiden: Brill. 45–72.

Clarke M. 1999, *Flesh and spirit in the songs of Homer*. Oxford: Clarendon Press.

Commager Jr. H.S. 1957, 'Lucretius' interpretation of the plague' in *Harvard Studies in Classical Philology*. 62: 105–8.

Contino S. 2000, 'Osservazioni critico-letterarie sul *De medicina* di Celso' in *Les textes médicaux latins comme littérature: actes du VIe colloque international*

Bibliography

sur les textes médicaux latins (Nantes, 1–3 September 1998). Edit. A. Pigeaud and J. Pigeaud. Nantes: Université de Nantes. 46–52.

Cooke A. 2015, *Understanding psychosis and schizophrenia. A report by the Division of Clinical Psychology.* The British Psychological Society. Canterbury: Christ Church University.

Craik E.M. 2015, *The 'Hippocratic' corpus, content and context.* Oxon: Routledge.

Craik E.M. 2018, 'The Hippocratic question' in *The Cambridge companion to Hippocrates.* Edit. P. E. Portmann. Cambridge: Cambridge University Press. 25–37.

Cross J.R. 2018, *Hippocratic oratory: the poetics of early Greek medical prose.* Oxon: Routledge.

Dean-Jones L. 2003, 'Literacy and the charlatan in ancient Greek medicine' in *Written texts and the rise of literate culture in ancient Greece.* Edit. H. Yunis. Cambridge: Cambridge University Press. 97–121.

Debru A. 1982, 'L'epilepsie dans le *De somno* d'Aristote' in *Médecins et médecine dans l'Antiquité: actes des Journées d'étude sur la médecine antique d'époque romaine* (Saint-Étienne, 14–15 mai 1982). Edit. G. Sabbah. Saint-Étienne: Université de Saint-Étienne. 25–41.

Devinant J. 2020, *Les troubles psychiques selon Galien.* Paris: Les belles lettres.

di Benedetto V. 1986, *Il medico e la malattia: la scienza di Ippocrate.* Torino: Enaudi.

Donini P. 1988, 'The history of the concept of eclecticism' in *The question of 'Eclecticism', Studies in later Greek philosophy.* Edit. J.M. Dillon and A. A. Long. Berkley and Los Angeles: University of California Press. 15–34.

Dossey L. 2013, 'Watchful Greeks and lazy Romans: Disciplining sleep in late antiquity' in *Journal of Early Christian Studies* 21(2): 209–39.

Flemming R. 2000, *Medicine and the making of Roman women: gender, nature and authority from Celsus to Galen.* Oxford: Oxford University Press.

Flemming R. 2012, 'Antiochus and Asclepiades: medical and philosophical sectarianism at the end of the Hellenistic era' in *The philosophy of Antiochus.* Edit. D. Sedley. Cambridge: Cambridge University Press. 55–79. http://access medicine.mhmedical.com/content.aspx?bookid=331&sectionid=40726737 (last accessed 30 June 2018).

Fögen T. 2009, *Wissen, Kommunikation und Selbstdarstellung: zur Struktur und Charakteristik römischer Fachtexte der frühen Kaiserzeit.* Munich: Beck.

Forster M. 2010, 'Wittgenstein on family resemblance concepts' in *Wittgenstein's philosophical investigations: A critical guide.* Edit. A. Ahmed. Cambridge: Cambridge University Press. 66–87.

Frede M. 1987, *Essays in ancient philosophy.* Minneapolis: University of Minnesota Press.

Freeman R. 2011, 'Chapter 20: Syncope' in *Harrison's principles of internal medicine.* 18th Ed. Edit. D.L. Longo, A.S. Fauci, D.L. Kasper, S.L. Hauser, J. L. Jameson and J. Loscalzo. USA: McGraw Hill. Online version.

Bibliography

Fulford K.W.M. 2006, *Oxford textbook of philosophy and psychiatry*. Oxford: Oxford University Press.

García Ballester L. 1997, 'Introducción' in *Sobre la localización de las enfermedades*. Translated by Salud Andrés Aparicio. Madrid: Gredos.

Garofalo I. 1988, *Erasistrati fragmenta*. Pisa: Giardini.

Garofalo I. 1997, *Anonymi medici de morbis acutis et chroniis*. Leiden: Brill.

Gautherie A. 2017, *Rhétorique et thérapeutique dans le De medicina de Celse*. Turnhout: Brepols Publishers.

Gill C. 2009, 'Psychology' in *The Cambridge companion to Epicureanism*. Edit. J. Warren. Cambridge: Cambridge University Press. 125–41.

Gould R. 2014, 'Antiquarianism as genealogy: Arnaldo Momigliano's method' in *History and Theory* 53: 212–33.

Gourevitch D. 1983, 'L'aphonie hippocratique' in *Formes de pensée dans la collection hippocratique: actes du IVe colloque international hippocratique* (Lausanne, 21–26 September 1981). Edit. F. Lasserre and P. Mudry. Geneva: Librairie Droz. 297–305.

Gourevitch D. 1991, 'Les mots pour dire la folie en latin. À propos de passages de Celse et de Célius Aurélien' in *L'Evolution Psychiatrique* 56(3): 561–8.

Gourevitch D and Grmek M.D. 1994, 'Aux sources de la doctrine médicale de Galien: l'enseignement de Marinus, Quintus et Numisianus' in *ANRW* 37.II: 1491–528.

Grmek M.D. 1983, *Les maladies à l'aube de la civilisation occidentale: recherches sur la réalité pathologique dans le monde grec préhistorique, archaïque et classique*. Paris: Payot.

Gundert B. 2000, 'Soma and psyche in Hippocratic medicine' in *Psyche and soma: physicians and metaphysicians on the mind–body problem from antiquity to Enlightenment*. Edit. J.P. Wright and P. Potter. Oxford: Clarendon. 13–35.

Hankinson R.J. 1991, 'Greek medical models of mind' in *Psychology*. Edit. S. Everson. Cambridge: Cambridge University Press. 194–217.

Hankinson R.J. 2006, 'Body and soul in Galen' in *Common to body and soul: philosophical approaches to explaining living behaviour in Greco-Roman antiquity*. Ed. R.A.H. King. Berlin: De Gruyter.

Hankinson R.J. 2008, 'The man and his work' in *The Cambridge companion to Galen*. Ed. R. J. Hankinson. Cambridge: Cambridge University Press.

Harris W.V. 2009, *Dreams and experience in classical antiquity*. Cambridge, MA: Harvard University Press.

Harris W.V. 2013a, *Mental disorders in the classical world*. Edit. W.V. Harris. Leiden and Boston: Brill.

Harris W.V. 2013b, 'Greek and Roman hallucinations' in *Mental disorders in the classical world*. Edit. W.V. Harris. Leiden and Boston: Brill. 285–306.

Hatzimichali M. 2011, *Potamo of Alexandria and the emergence of Eclecticism in late Hellenistic philosophy*. Cambridge: Cambridge University Press.

Bibliography

Hellweg R. 1985, *Stilistische Untersuchungen zu den Krankengeschichten der Epidemienbücher I und III des Corpus Hippocraticum.* Bonn: Habelt.

Holmes B. 2010, *The symptom and the subject.* Princeton, NJ: Princeton University Press.

Holmes B. 2013, 'Disturbing connections: sympathetic affections, mental disorder, and the elusive soul in Galen' in *Mental disorders in the classical world.* Ed. W.V. Harris. Leiden: Brill. 147–76.

Hüffmeier F. 1961, 'Phronesis in den Schriften des Corpus Hippocraticum' in *Hermes* 89(1): 51–84.

Hugues J.C. 2013, 'If only the ancients had had the DSM all would have been crystal clear: reflections on diagnosis' in *Mental disorders in the classical world.* Edit. W.V. Harris. Leiden and Boston: Brill. 41–58.

Hulskamp M.A.A. 2013, 'The value of dream diagnosis in the medical praxis of the Hippocratics and Galen' in *Dreams, healing, and medicine in Greece.* Edit. S.V. Oberhelman. New York and London: Routledge. Accessed online version: https://www.worldcat.org/title/dreams-healing-and-medicine-in-greece-from-antiquity-to-the-present/oclc/952727798/ viewport (last accessed 1 November 2019).

Hünenmörder C. 'Beaver' in *Brill's New Pauly Online*: https://referenceworks-brillonline.com.ezp.lib.cam.ac.uk/search?s.f.s2_parent=s.f.book.brill-s-new-pauly&search-go=&s.q=Beaver (last accessed 17 November 2019).

Johnston I. 2006, *Galen, on diseases and symptoms.* Cambridge: Cambridge University Press.

Jones W.H.S. 1923, *Hippocrates Vol. 2 On the sacred disease.* Cambridge, MA: Harvard University Press.

Jones W.H.S. 1931, *Hippocrates Vol. 4 On regimen.* Cambridge, MA: Harvard University Press.

Josephson S.A. and Miller B.L. 2018, 'Chapter 24: Confusion and delirium' in *Harrison's principles of internal medicine.* 20th Ed. Edit. by D.L. Longo, A. S. Fauci, D.L. Kasper, S.L. Hauser, J.L. Jameson and J. Loscalzo. USA: McGraw Hill. Online version: https://accessmedicine.mhmedical.com/content.aspx?sectionid=192011608&bookid=2129&Resultclick=2#1160872254 (last accessed 8 October 2019).

Jouanna J. 1983, 'Le sommeil médecin' in *Théâtre et spectacles dans l'Antiquité* (Actes du colloque de Strasbourg, novembre 1981). Leiden: Brill. 49–62.

Jouanna J. 1999, *Hippocrates.* Baltimore: Johns Hopkins University Press.

Jouanna J. 2012, 'Galen's reading of the Hippocratic treatise the *Nature of man*: the foundations of Hippocratism in Galen' in *Greek medicine from Hippocrates to Galen: selected papers.* Edit. P. van der Eijk. Leiden: Brill. 313–34.

Jouanna J. 2013, 'The typology and aetiology of madness in ancient Greek medical and philosophical writing' in *Mental disorders in the classical world.* Edit. by W.V. Harris. Leiden and Boston: Brill. 97–118.

Bibliography

King H. 2006, 'Introduction' in *Common to body and soul: philosophical approaches to explaining living behaviour in Greco-Roman antiquity*. Edit. R.A.H. King. Berlin: De Gruyter.

König J. and Woolf G. 2013, 'Encyclopaedism in the Roman Empire' in *Encyclopaedism from antiquity to the Renaissance*. Edit. J. König and G. Woolf. Cambridge: Cambridge University Press. 23–63.

Laes C. 2018, *Disabilities and the disabled in the Roman world: a social and cultural history*. Cambridge: Cambridge University Press.

Lakoff G. 1987, *Women, fire and dangerous things: what categories reveal about the mind*. Chicago: University of Chicago Press.

Lang P. 2013, *Medicine and society in Ptolemaic Egypt*. Leiden: Brill.

Langslow D.R. 1994, 'Celsus and the makings of Latin medical terminology' in *La médecine de Celse: aspects historiques, scientifiques et littéraires*. Edit. G. Sabbah and P. Mudry. Saint-Étienne: Publications de l'Université de Saint-Étienne. 297–309.

Langslow D.R. 2000, *Medical Latin in the Roman Empire*. Oxford: Oxford University Press.

Laskaris J. 2002, *The art is long: on the sacred disease and the scientific tradition*. Leiden, Boston and Köln: Brill.

Laureys S. 2007 'Eyes open, brain shut' in *Scientific American*. May: 32–7.

Leith D. 2009, 'The qualitative status of the *onkoi* in Asclepiades' theory of matter' in *Oxford studies in ancient philosophy*. Oxford: Oxford University Press. 283–320.

Leith D. 2015, 'Erasistratus' *triplokia* of arteries veins and nerves' in *Apeiron*. 48(3): 251–62.

Lewis O. 2018, 'Archigenes of Apamea's treatment of mental diseases' in *Mental illness in ancient medicine: from Celsus to Paul of Aegina*. Edit. C. Thumiger and P. Singer. Leiden: Brill. 143–75.

Lloyd G.E.R. 1983, *Science, folklore and ideology: studies in the life sciences in ancient Greece*. Cambridge: Cambridge University Press.

Longrigg J. 1989, 'Anatomy in Alexandria in the third century B.C.' in *British Journal of the History of Science* 21: 455–88.

Longrigg J. 1993, *Greek rational medicine: philosophy and medicine from Alcmaeon to the Alexandrians*. London: Routledge.

Lonie I.A. 1981, *The Hippocratic treatises 'On generation', 'On the nature of the child', 'Diseases IV' a commentary*. Berlin: De Gruyter.

Lonie I.A. 1983, 'Literacy and the development of Hippocratic medicine' in *Formes de pensée dans la collection hippocratique: actes du IVe colloque international hippocratique* (Lausanne, 21–26 September 1989). Edit. F. Lasserre and P. Mudry. Geneva: Librairie Droz. 145–61.

Lopez Morales D. 1999, 'Dos interpretaciones de la anormalidad psíquica: *Vict.* 35 y *Morb. Sacr.* 15' in *Le normal et le pathologique dans la collection hippocratique: actes du Xe colloque hippocratique* (Nice, 6–9 October 1999).

Bibliography

Edit. A. Thivel and A. Zucker. Nice-Sophia Antipolis: Publications de la Faculté des Lettres, Arts et Sciences humaines. 309–21.

López Salvá M. 1999, 'Efectos patológicos del vino en el corpus Hippocraticum' in *Le normal et le pathologique dans la collection hippocratique: actes du Xe colloque hippocratique* (Nice, 6–9 October 1999). Edit. A. Thivel and A. Zucker. Nice-Sophia Antipolis: Publications de la Faculté des Lettres, Arts et Sciences humaines. 523–37.

Lo Presti R. 2013, 'Mental disorder and the perils of definition: characterizing epilepsy in Greek scientific discourse (5th–4th centuries BCE)' in *Mental disorders in the classical world*. Edit. W.V. Harris. Leiden and Boston: Brill. 195–222.

Marelli C. 1983, 'Place de la collection *Hippocratique* dans les theories biologiques sur le sommeil' in *Formes de pensée dans la collection hippocratique: actes du IVe colloque international hippocratique* (Lausanne, 21–26 September 1981). Edit. F. Lasserre and P. Mudry. Geneva: Librairie Droz. 331–9.

Martinez Conesa J.A. 1974, 'La fenomenología del sueño en Celso' in *Durius* 2: 67–78.

Matentzoglu S. 2011, Zur Psychopathologie in den hippokratischen Schriften. Friedrich-Alexander-Universität Erlangen-Nürnberg: PhD dissertation.

Mattern S. 2008, *Galen and the rhetoric of healing*. Baltimore: Johns Hopkins University Press.

Mattern S. 2013, *The prince of medicine: Galen in the Roman Empire*. Oxford: Oxford University Press.

Mazzini I. 1992, 'Ippocrate in Celso' in *Tratados hipocráticos: estudios acerca de su contenido, forma e influencia (actas del VIIe colloque international hippocratique 24–29 Sept. 1990, Madrid)*. Edit. J.A. López Férez. Madrid: Universidad Nacional de Educación a Distancia. 571–83.

McDonald G.C. 2009a, Concepts and treatments of *phrenitis* in ancient medicine. University of Newcastle: PhD dissertation.

McDonald G.C. 2009b, 'Mapping madness: two medical responses to insanity in later antiquity' in *Acta Classica: Proceedings of the Classical Association of South Africa*. Supplementum 3: 106–29.

McDonald G.C. 2011, 'The body and space the *locus affectus* in ancient medical theories of disease' in *Medicine and space: body, surroundings and borders in antiquity and the Middle Ages*. Edit. P.A. Baker, H. Nijdam and K. van Land. Leiden: Brill. 61–83.

McDonald G.C. 2014, 'Galen on mental illness: a physiological approach to *phrenitis*' in *Philosophical themes in Galen*. Edit. P. Adamson, R. Hansberger and J. Wilberding. London: Institute of Classical Studies, School of Advanced Study, University of London. 135–53.

Momigliano A. 1950, 'Ancient history and the antiquarian' in *Journal of the Warburg and Courtauld Institutes*, Vol. 13, No. 3/4: 285–315.

Mudry P. 1993, 'L'orientation doctrinale du *De medicina* de Celse' in *ANRW II* 37.1. Berlin and New York: De Gruyter. 800–18.

Bibliography

Mudry P. 1994, 'Maladies graves et maladies mortelles. Présence et évolution d'une notion hippocratique chez les auteurs médicaux latins et en particulier Celse' in *Tradición e innovación de la medicina latina de la Antigüedad y de la Alta Edad Media: actas del IV coloquio internacional sobre los 'textos médicos latinos antiguos'*. Edit M.E. Vázquez Buján. Santiago de Compostela: Servicio de Publicacións e Intercambio Científico da Universidade de Santiago de Compostela. 133–43.

Mudry P. 2006a, 'Pour une rhetorique de la description des maladies. L'example de la médecine de Celse' in *Medicina, soror philosophiae: regards sur la littérature et les textes médicaux antiques (1975–2005)*. Edit. B. Maire. Lausanne: Editions BHMS. 9–18.

Mudry P. 2006b, 'Réflexions sur la medicine romaine' in *Medicina, soror philosophiae: regards sur la littérature et les textes médicaux antiques (1975–2005)*. Edit. B. Maire. Lausanne: Editions BHMS. 397–408.

Mudry P. 2006c, 'Maladies graves et maladies mortelles. Présence et évolution d'une notion hippocratique chez les auteurs médicaux latins et en particulier Celse' in *Medicina, soror philosophiae: regards sur la littérature et les textes médicaux antiques (1975–2005)*. Edit. B. Maire. Lausanne: Editions BHMS. 133–43.

Murphy E.A. 2013, The conceptualization and treatments for phrenitis, mania and melancholia in Aretaeus of Cappadocia and Caelius Aurelianus. University of Calgary: PhD dissertation.

Nagel T. 1974, 'What is it like to be a bat?' in *Philosophical Review* 83: 435–50.

Nissin L. 2016, *Roman sleep: sleeping areas and sleeping arrangements in the Roman house*. Helsinki: University of Helsinki.

Nutton V. 1995, 'Roman medicine 250 BC to AD 200' in *The western medical tradition*. Edit. L.I. Conrad, M. Neve, V. Nutton, R. Potter and A. Wear. Cambridge: Cambridge University Press.

Nutton V. 2008, 'Rufus of Ephesus in the medical context of his time' in *On melancholy, Rufus of Ephesus*. Edit. by Peter E. Pormann. Tübingen: Mohr Siebeck. 139–58.

Nutton V. 2013a, *Ancient medicine*. 2nd Ed. London: Routledge.

Nutton V. 2013b, 'Galenic madness' in *Mental disorders in the classical world*. Ed. W.V. Harris. Leiden: Brill. 119–27.

Oberhelman S.M. 1993, 'On the chronology and Pneumatism of Aretaios of Cappadocia' in *ANRW II* 37.2. Berlin and New York: De Gruyter. 941–66.

Oberhelman S.M. 2016, 'Introduction: medical pluralism, healing, and dreams in Greek culture' in *Dreams, healing, and medicine in Greece: from antiquity to the present*. Edit. S.M. Oberhelman. Routledge. 15–50.

Padel R. 1994, *In and out of the mind: Greek images of the tragic self*. Princeton, NJ: Princeton University Press.

Pardon M. 2005, 'Celsus and the *Hippocratic corpus*: the originality of a plagiarist' in *Hippocrates in context: papers read at the XIth international*

Bibliography

Hippocrates colloquium (University of Newcastle upon Tyne, 2002). Edit. P. J. van der Eijk. Leiden: Brill. 403–11.

Pelavski A. 2020, 'Questioning the obvious: the use of questions and answers in assessing consciousness in the Hippocratic corpus' in *Ancient Greek medicine in questions and answers*. Edit. M. Meeusen. Leiden: Brill. 8–27.

Pelavski A. 2023, 'Impaired consciousness, madness and mental incapacitation in the Roman law' in *Classical World*. 116.4: 399–426.

Perez Molina M.E. 1998, *Areteo de Cappadocia, Obra médica*. Madrid: Ediciones Akal.

Perrilli L. 2018, 'Epistemologies' in *The Cambridge companion to Hippocrates*. Edit. P. E. Portmann. Cambridge: Cambridge University Press. 119–51.

Petit C. 2009, *Galien., le médecin* (Vol. 3). Edit., introduced and translated by C. Petit. Paris: Les belles lettres.

Pigeaud J. 1981, *La maladie de l'âme: étude sur la relation de l'âme et du corps dans la tradition médico-philosophique antique*. Paris: Les belles lettres.

Pigeaud, J. 1987, *Folie et cures de la folie chez les médecins de l'antiquité gréco-romaine. La manie*. Paris: Les belles lettres.

Pigeaud J. 1994, 'La reflexion de Celse sur la folie' in *La médecine de Celse: aspects historiques, scientifiques et littéraires*. Edit. G. Sabbah and P. Mudry. Saint-Étienne: Publications de l'Université de Saint-Étienne. 257–79.

Pigeaud, J. 2004, 'La rhétorique d'Arétée' in *La médecine grecque antique: actes du 14ème colloque de la Villa Kérylos* (Beaulieu-sur-Mer 10–11 October 2003). Cahiers de la Villa de Kerylos n. 15, Edit. J. Leclant and J. Jouanna. Paris: Académie des Inscriptions et Belles-Lettres. 177–97.

Pigeaud J. 2008, *Poetiques du corps*. Paris: Les belles lettres.

Polansky R. 2007, *Aristotle's De anima*. Cambridge: Cambridge University Press.

Polito R. 2006, 'Matter, medicine and the mind: Asclepiades vs. Epicurus' in *Oxford Studies in Ancient Philosophy*. Oxford: Oxford University Press. 285–335.

Rao K.R. 1998, 'Two faces of consciousness: a look at eastern and western perspectives' in *Journal of Consciousness Studies*, 5(3), 309–27.

Rawson E. 1985, *Intellectual life in the late Roman Republic*. London: Duckworth.

Renberg G. 2017, *Where dreams may come: incubation sanctuaries in the Greco-Roman world*. Leiden: Brill.

Rocca J. 2003, *Galen on the brain: anatomical knowledge and physiological speculation on the second century AD*. Leiden: Brill.

Rodriguez Alfageme I. 1999, 'Patología del habla en el *corpus Hippocraticum*' in *Le normal et le pathologique dans la collection hippocratique: actes du Xe colloque hippocratique* (Nice, 6–9 October 1999). Edit. A. Thivel and A. Zucker. Nice-Sophia Antipolis: Publications de la Faculté des Lettres, Arts et Sciences humaines. 149–71.

Bibliography

Rosch E. 1975, 'Cognitive representation of semantic categories' in *Journal of Experimental Psychology: General*. 104: 192–233.

Roselli A. 2004, 'Les malades d'Arétée de Cappadoce' in *La médecine grecque antique: actes du 14ème colloque de la Villa Kérylos* (Beaulieu-sur-Mer 10–11 October 2003). Cahiers de la Villa de Kerylos n. 15, Edit. J. Leclant and J. Jouanna. Paris: Académie des Inscriptions et Belles-Lettres. 163–76.

Sanders R.D., Tononi G., Laureys S. and Sleigh J. 2012, 'Unresponsiveness ≠ unconsciousness' in *Anesthesiology* 116(4): 946–59.

Scarborough J. 1993, 'Roman medicine to Galen' in *ANRW* II 37.1. Berlin and New York: De Gruyter. 3–58.

Schneider U.J. 1998, 'Eclecticism rediscovered' in *Journal of the History of Ideas*. 59.1: 173–82.

Schöner E. 1964, 'Das Vierschema in der antiken Humoralpathologie' in *Sudhoffs Arch. f. Gesch. d. Med*. Suppl. 4. Wiesbaden: Steiner.

Seeley W.W. and Miller B.L. 2018, 'Chapter 25: Dementia' in *Harrison's principles of internal medicine*. 20th Ed. Edit. by D.L. Longo, A.S. Fauci, D. L. Kasper, S.L. Hauser, J.L. Jameson and J. Loscalzo. USA: McGraw Hill. Online version: http://accessmedicine.mhmedical.com/content.aspx?book id=331&sectionid=40726737 (last accessed 8 October 2019).

Servat G. 1995, *Celse: De la médecine. Livres I et II*. Paris: Les belles lettres.

Shields C. 2018, 'Theories of mind in the Hellenistic period' in *A history of mind and body in late antiquity*. Edit. A. Marmodoro and S. Cartwright. Cambridge: Cambridge University Press. 33–51.

Siegel R.E. 1973, *Galen on psychology, psychopathology, and function and diseases of the nervous system; an analysis of his doctrines, observations and experiments*. Basel and New York: Karger.

Simon B. 2013, 'Carving the nature at the joints': the dream of a perfect classification of mental illness' in *Mental disorders in the classical world*. Edit. W.V. Harris. Leiden and Boston: Brill. 27–40.

Singer P.N. 1992, 'Some Hippocratic mind–body problems' in *Tratados hipocráticos: estudios acerca de su contenido, forma e influencia – actas del VIIe colloque international hippocratique* (Madrid, 24–29 September 1990). Edit. J.A. Lopez Ferez. Madrid: Universidad Nacional de Educación a Distancia. 131–43.

Singer P.N. 2013, *Galen psychological writings*. Cambridge: Cambridge University Press.

Smith W.D. 1979, *The Hippocratic tradition*. Ithaca, NY and London: Cornell University Press.

Stahl W.H. 1962, *Roman science: origins, development, and influence to the later Middle Ages*. Madison: University of Wisconsin Press.

Stannard J. 1964, 'Materia medica and philosophic theory in Aretaeus' in *Sudhoffs Archiv für Geschichte der Medizin und der Naturwissenschaften*: Bd. 48, H. 1: 27–53.

Bibliography

Stok F. 1993, 'La medicina nell'enciclopedia latina e nei sistemi di classificazione delle arti dell'età romana' in *ANRW II* 37.1. Berlin and New York: De Gruyter. 393–444.

Stok F. 1996, 'Follia e malattie mentali nella medicina dell'età romana' in *ANRW II* 37.3. Berlin and New York: De Gruyter. 2283–365.

Stok F. 2010, 'Cicerone e la politica del sogno' in *Sub imagine somni: nighttime phenomena in Greco-Roman culture*. Edit. E. Scioli and C. Walde. Pisa: ETS. 103–18.

Strobl P. 2002, *Die Macht des Schlafes in der Griechisch-Römischen Welt. Eine Untersuchung der mythologischen und physiologischen Aspekte der antiken Standpunkte*. Hamburg: Kovac.

Taylor B. 1993, 'Unconsciousness and society: The sociology of sleep' in *International Journal of Politics, Culture and Society*. 6 (3): 463–71.

Teasdale G. and Jennet B. 1974, 'Assessment of coma and impaired consciousness: a practical scale' in *The Lancet* 2: 81–4.

Teasdale G., Maas A., Lecky F., Manley G., Stocchetti N. and Murray G. 2014, 'The Glasgow Coma Scale at 40 years: standing the test of time' in *The Lancet* 13: 844–52.

Thorarinsdottir E.H., Bjornsdottir E., Benediktsdottir B., Janson C., Gislason T., Aspelund T., Kuna S.T., Pack A.I. and Arnardottir E.S. 2019, 'Definition of excessive daytime sleepiness in the general population: feeling sleepy relates better to sleep-related symptoms and quality of life than the Epworth sleepiness scale score. Results from an epidemiological study' in *Journal of Sleep Research* 28: Dec(6). e12852.

Thumiger C. 2013, 'The early Greek medical vocabulary of insanity' in *Mental disorders in the classical world*. Edit. W.V. Harris. Leiden and Boston: Brill. 61–95.

Thumiger C. 2017, *A history of the mind and mental health in classical Greek medical thought*. Cambridge: Cambridge University Press.

Tieleman T. 2003, 'Galen's psychology' in *Galien et la philosophie: huit exposés suivis de discussions*. Edit. J. Barnes and J. Jouanna. Geneva: Fondation Hardt. 131–70.

Tracy T.J. 1976, 'Plato, Galen, and the center of consciousness' in *Illinois Classical Studies* 1: 43–52.

Tranel D. 2003, 'Higher brain functions' in *Neuroscience in medicine*. Edit. P.M. Conn. Totowa, NJ: Humana Press Inc. 651–66.

Vallance J.T. 1990, *The lost theory of Asclepiades of Bythinia*. Oxford: Oxford University Press.

van der Eijk P.J. 1997, 'Towards a rhetoric of ancient scientific discourse: some formal characteristics of Greek medical and philosophical texts (Hippocratic Corpus, Aristotle)' in *Grammar as interpretation*. Edit. E.J. Bakker. Leiden: Brill. 77–129.

van der Eijk P.J. 1999, 'The *Anonymus Parisinus* and the doctrines of the ancients' in *Ancient histories of medicine: essays in medical doxography and*

Bibliography

historiography in classical antiquity. Edit. P. J. van der Eijk. Leiden: Brill. 295–331.

van der Eijk P.J. 2005, *Medicine and philosophy in classical antiquity: doctors and philosophers on nature, soul, health and disease*. Edit. P.J. van der Eijk. Cambridge: Cambridge University Press. 119–35.

van der Eijk P.J. 2013, 'Cure and (in)curability of mental disorders in ancient medical and philosophical thought' in *Mental disorders in the classical world*. Edit. W.V. Harris. Leiden: Brill. 307–38.

Vazquez Buján M.E. 1988, 'Réception latine de quelques concepts médicaux grecs' in *Études de médecine romaine (Mémoirs VIII)*. Edit. G. Sabbah. Saint-Étienne: Université de Saint-Étienne. 167–75.

Verbeke G. 1945, *L'évolution de la doctrine du pneuma du stoïcisme à saint Augustin. Étude philosophique*. Paris: D. de Brouwe.

Verde F. 2020, 'The partition of the soul in Epicurus, Demetrius Lacon and Diogenes of Oinoanda' in *Body and soul in Hellenistic philosophy*. Edit. B. Inwood and J. Warren. Cambridge: Cambridge University Press. 89–112.

von Staden H. 1982, '*Hairesis* and heresy: the case of the *haireseis iatrikai*' in *Jewish and Christian self-definition, III: Self-definition in the Greco-Roman world*. Edit. B.F. Meyer and E.P Sanders. London: SCM Press. 199–206.

von Staden H. 1989, *Herophilus: the art of medicine in early Alexandria, edition, translation and essays*. Cambridge: Cambridge University Press.

von Staden H. 1994a, 'Author and authority: Celsus and the construction of a scientific self' in *Tradición e innovación de la medicina latina de la Antigüedad y de la Alta Edad Media: actas del IV coloquio internacional sobre los 'textos médicos latinos antiguos'*. Edit M.E. Vázquez Buján. Santiago de Compostela: Servicio de Publicacións e Intercambio Científico da Universidade de Santiago de Compostela. 103–17.

von Staden H. 1994b, '*Media quodammodo diuersas inter sententias*: Celsus, the 'rationalists', and Erasistratus' in *La médecine de Celse: aspects historiques, scientifiques et littéraires*. Edit. G. Sabbah and P. Mudry. Saint-Étienne: Publications de l'Université de Saint-Étienne. 77–101.

von Staden H. 1997, 'Galen and the Second Sophistic' in *Bulletin of the Institute of Classical Studies* 41, 68(supp): 33–54.

von Staden H. 1999, 'Celsus as historian?' in *Ancient histories of medicine: essays in medical doxography and historiography in classical antiquity*. Edit. P. J. van der Eijk. Leiden: Brill. 251–94.

von Staden H. 2000, 'The dangers of literature and the need for literacy: A. Cornelius Celsus on reading and writing' in *Les textes médicaux latins comme littérature: actes du VIe colloque international sur les textes médicaux latins* (Nantes, 1–3 September 1998). Edit. A. Pigeaud and J. Pigeaud. Nantes: Université de Nantes. 355–68.

von Staden H. 2002, 'Body, soul, and nerves: Epicurus, Herophilus, Erasistratus, the Stoics, and Galen' in *Psyche and soma: physicians and metaphysicians on*

Bibliography

the mind–body problem from antiquity to Enlightenment. Edit. J.P. Wright and P. Potter. Oxford: Clarendon Press. 79–116.

von Staden H. 2010, 'How Greek was the Latin body? The parts and the whole in Celsus' *Medicina*' in *Body, disease and treatment in a changing world: Latin texts and contexts in ancient and medieval medicine. Proceedings of the ninth international conference 'Ancient Latin medical texts*' (University of Manchester, September 2007). Edit. D. Langslow and B. Maire. Lausanne: Éditions BHMS. 3–23.

Wallace-Hadrill A. 2008, *Rome's cultural revolution*. Cambridge: Cambridge University Press.

Walshe T.M. 2016, *Neurological concepts in ancient Greek medicine*. New York: Oxford University Press.

Webster C. 2016, 'Voice pathologies and the Hippocratic triangle', in *Homo patiens – Approaches to the patient in the ancient world*. Ed. G. Petridou and C. Thumiger. Leiden: Brill. 166–99.

Williams S.J. 2008, 'The sociological significance of sleep: progress, problems and perspectives' in *Sociology Compass* 2 (2): 639–43.

Worthman C.M. and Melby M.K. 2002, 'Toward a comparative developmental ecology of human sleep' in *Adolescent sleep patterns: biological, social, and psychological influences*. Edit. M.A. Carskadon. New York: Cambridge University Press. 69–117.

INDEX

Index

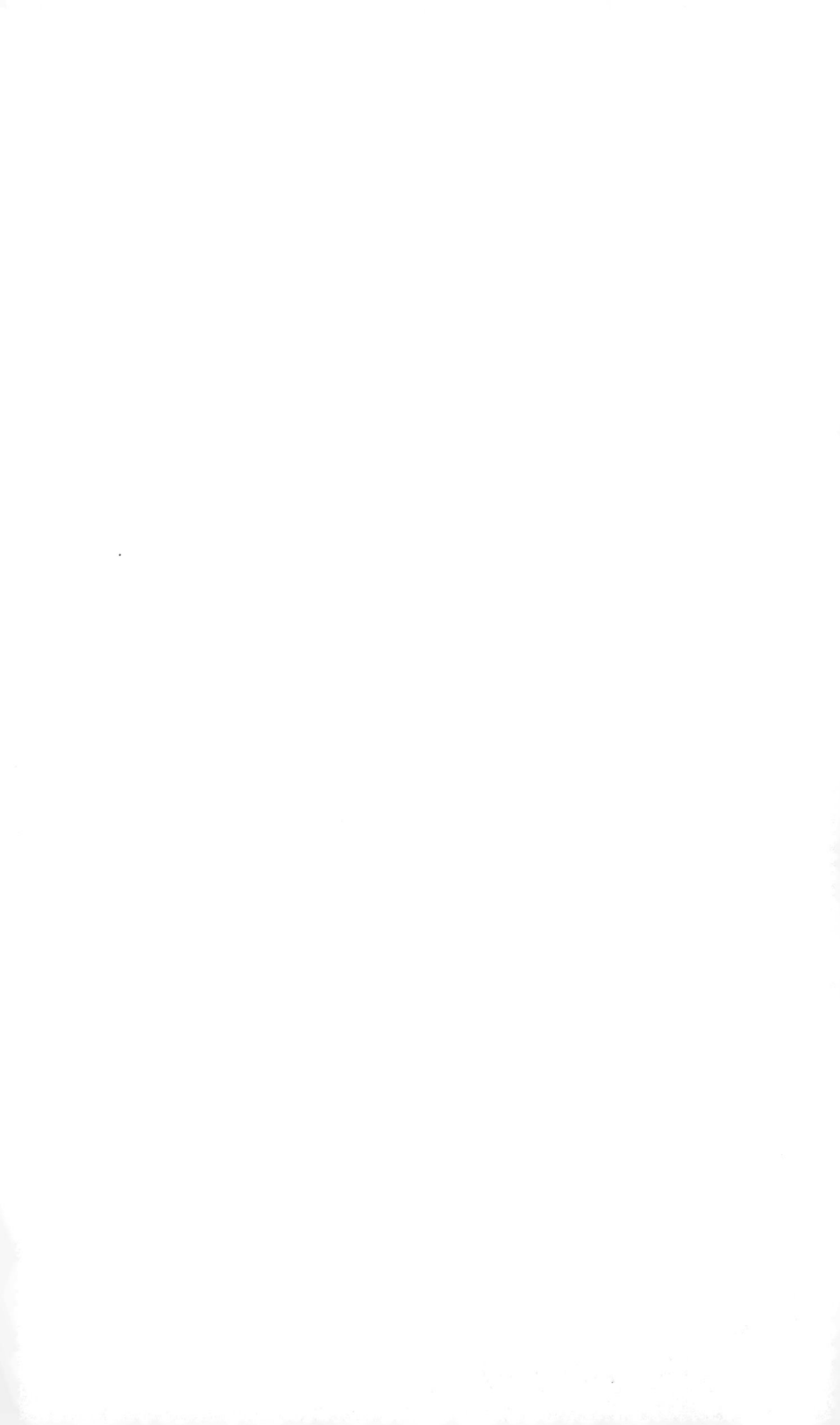

For EU product safety concerns, contact us at Calle de José Abascal, 56–1°, 28003 Madrid, Spain or eugpsr@cambridge.org.

www.ingramcontent.com/pod-product-compliance
Ingram Content Group UK Ltd.
Pitfield, Milton Keynes, MK11 3LW, UK
UKHW022008061225

465726UK00012B/482